Nursing leadership in action

PRINCIPLES AND APPLICATION TO STAFF SITUATIONS

LAURA MAE DOUGLASS
R.N., B.A., M.S.
Chairman, Division of Nursing, Point Loma
College, San Diego, California

EM OLIVIA BEVIS
R.N., B.S., M.A.
Professor of Nursing, California
State University, San Jose, California

SECOND EDITION

Saint Louis
THE C. V. MOSBY COMPANY 1974

SECOND EDITION

Copyright © 1974 by The C. V. Mosby Company

All rights reserved. No part of this book may be reproduced in any manner without written permission of the publisher.

First edition copyrighted 1970

Printed in the United States of America

Distributed in Great Britain by Henry Kimpton, London

Library of Congress Cataloging in Publication Data

Douglass, Laura Mae.
  Nursing leadership in action.

  Published in 1970 under title: Team leadership in action.
    1. Team nursing. 2. Nursing service administration.
I. Bevis, Em Olivia, joint author. II. Title.
[DNLM: 1. Leadership. 2. Nursing, Supervisory.
WY105 D737t 1974]
RT90.5.D64   1974   658.31'28   74-674
ISBN 0-8016-1436-8

VH/M/M   9   8   7   6   5   4

Preface

Many things have happened to nursing in the four years since this book was first published under the title *Team Leadership in Action*. Rapid changes are sweeping all of the health-related disciplines. Nursing is attempting to devise care delivery systems that will better meet the needs of health consumers in ways that provide continuity, comprehension, and quality. New practice modes are marked by autonomy, authority, and accountability. Nurses still practice some form of collaborative delivery system in most areas of the country, but more and more agencies and individuals are attempting to structure delivery systems that will provide the client with better services and the nurse with greater challenge and satisfaction. Consequently, this book has enlarged its focus from leadership in team nursing to the broader spectrum of leadership in nursing. The principles of leadership apply regardless of the specific nursing care delivery system in use at a given agency.

Schools and agencies that teach nursing leadership principles for utilization in nursing practice in any type of delivery mode will produce a more flexible and skilled nurse.

Except for the broadened focus of the book, the basic intent has not changed. The book still attempts to help nurses learn the functions that make the delivery of nursing care work. Leadership activities, whether used in team nursing, primary nursing, functional nursing, or case nursing, require the leadership skills discussed here. Every nurse practices leadership by the very nature of nursing, for decisions must be made and problems solved whether they concern one or many patients or one or many nurses.

Education of nurses has traditionally emphasized the study of knowledge and skills of patient care with the assumption that the graduate could function in a leadership role with a minimum of preparation. This preparation was expected to be provided by the employer, who in turn anticipated that the graduate would be able to function in a leadership capacity from the first day of employment with only brief orientation to agency routine and policy. Lack of sufficient leadership preparation has resulted in the nurse's frustration and disenchantment with leadership activities and in disillusionment on the part of the employer whose expectations have not been met. Efforts to remedy this situation are being exerted by individuals, schools of nursing, professional organizations, and employing institutions. This book is designed to assist in this effort.

One goal of nursing education is to teach the use of foresight. Anticipating the results of behaviors and the effective use of self requires the ability to predict outcomes and therefore to behave in a way that will produce desired results. This book is an initial attempt to elaborate a theoretical framework for staff nursing that will enable the nurse to mobilize all available resources for the benefit of those who are in need of health service. Other goals are to provide a body of knowledge that will supply a theoretical framework of administrative principles for use by the nurse-leader, to provide a practical method for utilization of these administrative principles in day-to-day nursing activities, and to promote a cognitive habit in the nurse practitioner that will transform the nurse utilizing these knowledges and methods into an effective leader. These objectives are met through a consideration of the staff nurse as a leader and the formulation and utilization of principles necessary for effective leadership.

A theoretical framework for the book presents the basic hypotheses upon which the book is based. Subsequent chapters deal with teaching-learning, communication, delegating authority, evaluating personnel, changing, and leadership.

No attempt has been made to cover the entire field of the subjects implied by the chapter headings. We have carefully selected material that we consider to be most useful to nurses. The book continues to be designed for use by students, staff nurses, supervisory staff, teachers, and independent nurse practitioners.

We are grateful to family, friends, and colleagues who gave their understanding, support, and time so that this book could be written. We are especially grateful to our students whose need inspired the book and whose studies helped us grow.

Laura Mae Douglass
Em Olivia Bevis

Contents

Appendix, 203

CHAPTER ONE

Theoretical framework for the nurse-leader

All nurses today function as leaders. Health agencies in every setting and of every type expect nurses to be leaders of patients, nursing teams, health teams, and community groups.

Leadership is a learned behavior pattern. To function effectively the nurse must acquire fundamental principles that make leadership a learned process rather than a series of duties described and listed in a policy manual. Principles of effective leadership and their use can be learned by both the student and the experienced nurse. The knowledge, skill, and experience of every nurse can be organized so that the quality of leadership ability is improved. The development of leadership ability may be achieved through:

1. Formulating principles of leadership based on a sound body of knowledge (input)
2. Utilizing these principles systematically to solve problems (operation)
3. Obtaining evaluative feedback (feedback)

Learning principles of leadership through the traditional cognitive methods is insufficient. The term "leadership" implies operations and behaviors; it implies interaction with people; therefore, the knowledge and skills of leadership must be acquired where people work together.

This chapter establishes the theoretical framework from which the remainder of the book derives its form and structure. Basically, the authors and readers must be able to meet on conceptual and theoretical common ground. John Stuart Mills' admonition, ". . . above all, to insist upon having the meaning of a word clearly understood before using it, and the meaning of a proposition before assenting to it,"* clearly bespeaks the obvious need to set about a simple but scholarly task. That task is one of coming to grips with key concepts and hypotheses (meanings and propositions) prior to elaborating ideas that are both consequences of and subsequent to those theoretical constructs. Meanings and propositions will be provided for leadership, for the nature of roles and role assumption, for theories generally, with particular emphasis upon predictive theories or predictive principles, and for problem solving and decision making.

---

*From Mills' inaugural address as Rector, University of St. Andrews, February 1, 1867.

LEADERSHIP

June Bailey and her associates at the University of California, San Francisco, defined leadership as follows:

> Leadership behavior is a set of actions which influence members of a group to move toward goal setting and goal attainment. Inherent in the actions are the functional and interactive variables of the task, the organizational structure, the external environment, and the characteristics of the leader and the follower, particularly the assumptions and values that are held by group members. Elements in the spectrum of leadership behavior are communication, information processing, problem solving, decision making, change, innovation, human relations, and initiating and structuring behaviors. Thus, leadership behavior is viewed as multidimensional, encompassing structure, processes, functions, and human relationships.*

Leadership can only be defined by the behaviors manifested by leaders or by role enactment. Leadership that is defined only by leadership characteristics becomes nonfunctional; in other words, characteristics alone cannot be operationalized. If, as is hypothesized, leadership is a learned behavior and therefore can be taught, then it follows that leadership must be defined in some way that makes it feasible to operationalize the definition. For this reason, Dr. Bailey's definition is a highly pragmatic one. Fig. 1 is a model of the interactive flow of the components of leadership as defined. Note the set of actions (processes), the organizational structure (human relationships), and the task (goal setting–goal attainment functions) are all placed within the context of the characteristics and values of the leader and the led, and all the foregoing are placed within the larger context of the external environment.

For convenience the components of leadership behaviors have been grouped and dealt with in this book in a variety of ways in appropriate places. Information processing, problem solving, and decision making are covered in this chapter on theoretical framework. The section is labeled problem solving–decision making and includes goal setting and goal attainment. Information processing encompasses problem solving and learning and is treated here as predictive principle formation. Even though information processing is a larger process than that of formulating predictive principles, the limitations of the book preclude inclusion of the whole subject.

Communications and human relationships and the use of these processes in such contexts as conferences and group dynamics are covered in Chapter 3; initiating and structuring behaviors are dealt with in Chapters 2 and 4; and change and innovation are discussed in Chapters 5 and 6. It becomes clear that the complete separation of processes into exclusive categories is an artificial and sometimes arbitrary division. Each of the processes listed as sets of actions in the definition are used interrelatedly with each other process. *Leadership, then, is the ability to use the processes of life to facilitate the movement of a person, a group, a family, or a community toward the establishing and attainment of a goal. Nursing leadership is the ability to use the processes of life to facilitate the movement of a person, a group, a family, or a community toward the establishing and attainment of goals pertaining to health.*

---

*From Bailey, J.: An operational definition of leadership. Unpublished paper.

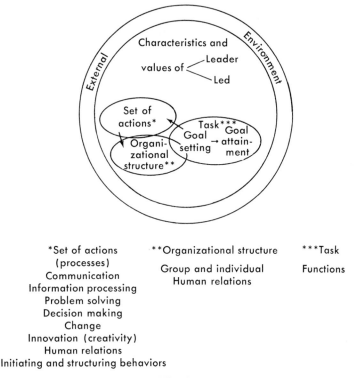

*Set of actions
(processes)
Communication
Information processing
Problem solving
Decision making
Change
Innovation (creativity)
Human relations
Initiating and structuring behaviors

**Organizational structure
Group and individual
Human relations

***Task
Functions

Fig. 1

PROCESS—A THEORY ABOUT THE NATURE OF THINGS

Inevitably, words must be used to define other words, and in the definition of leadership the words "process" and "processing" are used. The word "process" has become popular in education and in nursing during the last twenty years. People refer to *process* teaching, *processing* information, the *process* of problem solving, nursing *process*, and so on. One has but to connect the various ways the word is used and examine the context of its use to observe that the common denominator of meaning is flow, or, as Alfred North Whitehead labels it, flux.* Process is change toward an objective using feedback. Change—flow, flux, dynamics—is in the nature of all things. Some things flow more rapidly than others; the flow of time, measured by the rising and setting of the sun, is more rapid than the flow or change of granite. But even granite, that symbol of permanence, decomposes and crumbles; thus, it becomes part of the flux of nature.

Each change, each product of flux is new and unique from its antecedents; therefore, flux is the creative thrust of life. This creativity—uniqueness—comes about from the interaction and the mutually inclusive nature of processes. The result of interaction is that each process does indeed affect the "new" product. Take, for instance, the processes included in the definition of leadership. The

*Whitehead, A. N.: Process and reality, New York, 1929, The Macmillan Co.

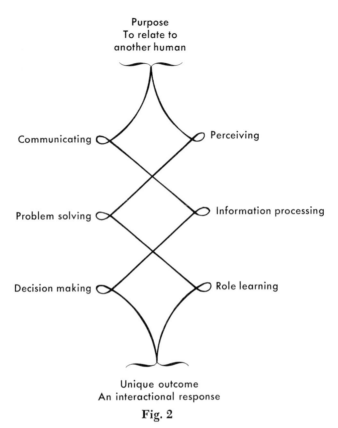

Fig. 2

process of relating to other humans includes elements of the process of communicating (see Fig. 2). One cannot communicate without processing information; for example, "to relate to" means (1) to perceive; (2) to validate, classify, sort, and interpret the perceptions (which is one way to process data); (3) to solve problems by thinking of alternative responses to the perceived messages; (4) to weigh the consequences of each possible response; and (5) to choose a response and respond to the other human being. Thus, in a single encounter in reacting to another human being, the processes of communication, information processing, problem solving, and decision making have all been used to initiate and structure one unique, new, transient act or behavior. Fig. 2 depicts how single processes interact, intertwine, and combine to produce a single new episode—a unique act or behavior. *A process has purpose, organization, and outcome. The purpose is the goal; the organization is the way in which many components or other processes unite to produce the unique outcome. The whole of the three components flow inexorably into the next life episode.*

One of the most common examples used to illustrate the nature of processes is the phenomenon of human reproduction. The purpose of reproduction is to continue the species. Each reproductive episode or successful birth produces a new, unique human being, different from any other human being; yet, siblings are created from the same antecedents or ancestors. The antecedents or ancestors combine in uniquely organized ways and provide endless alternative genetic combinations to produce an infinite number of possible products, or children—each child different from his sibling.

This concept of flux and flow and the unstoppable nature of this flow is beautifully expressed in the *Rubáiyát* of Omar Khayyám. The entire work is an expression of the flux of life. Captured in these few brief lines is part of that expression:

> The Moving Finger writes; and, having writ,
> Moves on: nor all your Piety nor Wit
>   Shall lure it back to cancel half a Line,
> Nor all your Tears wash out a Word of it.

The same idea is expressed in yet another short verse from the same work:

> YESTERDAY *This* Day's Madness did prepare;
> TO-MORROW's Silence, Triumph, or Despair:

A process, to summarize, is the phenomenon of life which hypothesizes that each thing has a purpose, an organization, and an innovative outcome, and that each innovative outcome is a result of many unique factors combining purposefully.

LEARNING THE LEADERSHIP ROLE

The leadership role, like any other role, is an organized set of behaviors assigned to a position. The behaviors become operational only when the position is occupied. The role of leader can be assumed when the position of leader is assumed. The leadership position can be attained by job description, by the power that knowledge and skill generate, by assumption of the role, or by investment of power by others. The leadership role is interactional in nature and cannot be learned or enacted out of the social context of complementary roles. In other words, every leader, to be a leader, must have someone, some group, to lead. The role of being led is the role that complements the role of leader. A leader not only must learn the leadership behaviors that enable the assumption of the leadership role, the leader must also learn the role of the led. Only through learning the complementary role of the led can a leader know and enact the leadership role appropriately.

A role is learned using an entire role set. The role set includes the role of *leader,* the *complementary role,* and the *audience* (interested others). The complementary role of the led creates the expectations of leadership behavior. Every patient who is led by a nurse has certain behavioral expectations for the nurse, which are communicated in overt and covert ways. The patient may communicate to the nurse-leader the expectation that the nurse will act as information giver, disciplinarian, nurturer or mother figure, authority person, teacher, decision maker, advocate or will display any number of other behaviors or functions. The better the nurse leader knows the complementary role of the led, the better the nurse will be able to perform the leadership role.

The audience, or interested others, performs vital functions, even though this group is neither the leader nor the led. For the nurse-leader role the audience may be families, supervisors, administrators, patients, or colleagues, depending upon who plays the complementary role of the led. For instance, if the patient is in the complementary role of the led, then families, supervisors, administrators, and the nurse's peers will be the audience. The audience performs the following functions: (1) creates the social reality of the role; (2) gives cues for leadership behaviors, expectations, and role enactment; (3) provides social reinforcement through praise, approval, participation, and rewards; and (4) contributes to the maintenance of the leadership role behavior.

Roles can be either ascribed or achieved. *Ascribed* roles are those roles people are born to or are granted through socialization. The roles of son, daughter, or child are examples of ascribed roles. These roles are attained through the process of socialization. *Achieved* roles, on the other hand, are roles one aspires to or earns. The role of nurse, for example, is an aspired role. One sets out to learn the nurse role; one sets out to learn the leader role. Achieved roles are more complex than ascribed roles in that they are superimposed on the ascribed role. Women nurses bring to the role learning of the nurse-leader characteristics and behaviors of the ascribed roles of women in this society—mother, daughter, sister. Similar superimposition of achieved role of nurse-leader on ascribed roles of men—father, brother, son—exists for men nurses.

One of the obvious problems of learning a professional role, such as nursing, is that role preconceptions of anticipatory socialization are simpler and more stereotyped than the reality of the role. The person aspiring to the role of nurse can envision a Sue Barton or a Cherry Ames, both highly stereotyped misconceptions of reality. Therefore, a conflict arises because preconceived role expectations do not conform to the complex reality of the role as it must be enacted. Further complications arise when previous learning of ascribed roles conflict with the learning needs of the achieved roles.

This pyramiding of roles (see Fig. 3) produces highly complex identity and behavioral learning situations. A clear picture of the various roles being played in one life episode enables the player to establish role priorities or role combinations compatible with role expectations of the audience and complementary role players.

One of the most useful skills in the nurse-leader's repertoire is the skill of role taking. Role taking is the ability to take on the role of another, to develop empathy, to adopt his view of the world, his attitudes, and to see problems and

Fig. 3

issues from his point of view. Role-taking behavior enables the leader to predict another's behavior and to develop his own behavior anticipatorially. Role taking facilitates healthy social interaction, a prime component of leadership behavior.

According to role theorists, roles must be learned as a Gestalt, or as a whole, total, organized pattern—including both the cognitive and behavorial components. Learning bits and pieces of a role can occur as separate learning episodes, but the success of role enactment is dependent upon the learner's ability to integrate the total set. In other words, learning of bits and pieces must be followed by learning of the interrelationship of these bits and pieces and insights and behaviors with the total field, or pattern. The implication of this statement for learning leadership roles is that leadership learning must occur in a manner that facilitates interaction, either real or simulated, with all characters, that is, leader, led, and audience. Learning each of these roles independently will not result in the ability to successfully enact the leadership role. Practice, with coaching, in situations in which all elements of the leadership set of behaviors occur is necessary for the leadership role to be achieved.

THEORIES—THE BASIS OF LEADERSHIP ACTIVITY*

A theory is an invention of man. Man theorizes to explain or speculate about what something is; what it is like, or what its characteristics and attributes are; how something exists in relation to other things; what circumstances or conditions will make things behave in certain ways, and what will prevent them from behaving in certain other ways; and, finally, how they can be used in life situations. In other words, a theory enables the nurse-leader to work with others in speculating about leadership problems, to devise hypotheses about alternative solutions to those problems, and to develop ways to test those hypotheses in nursing actions.

The word "theory" can be used in many different ways. People use "theory" to separate the cognitive components from the practical or activity components of a discipline. Sometimes "theory" is used to indicate the speculative as opposed to the proven; sometimes it is used to refer to guesses or hypotheses about how simpler concepts or laws relate to one another; sometimes it is used to mean predictions about how things are going to behave; and sometimes it is used to prescribe ways to make certain behaviors occur. "Theory" has so many definitions because it is a complex phenomenon, and all the definitions or meanings listed above do refer to one or more of its aspects (sometimes referred to as levels). Theories evolve through a hierarchy of serial levels. They are still theories, regardless of the level of development they are in. An analogy to this phenomenon of theory levels can be found in Erikson's theory of human development. Human development theory maintains that success in life or human maturity is attained when each central task of development is accomplished, at least in part, in its proper order. Further, full maturity is not attained until these

---

*This discussion on theory is adapted from Bevis, E. O.: Curriculum building in nursing: a process, St. Louis, 1973, The C. V. Mosby Co.; and derived and synthesized from the works of Dickoff, James, and Wiedenbach; Gagne; and Abdulla and Levine (see Bibliography).

tasks of development are minimally accomplished. In the same manner, the attainment of the highest level of theories is dependent upon the successful completion of each prior level of that theory. *Skilled leadership exploits a given theory or hypothesis by testing out in practice the validity of the prediction.*

The four levels or phases of theories in practice disciplines

Four stages of development are necessary for a theory to reach its full maturity and thus be optimally useful in nurse leadership practice. These theory levels are labeled (1) factor isolating, (2) factor relating, (3) situation relating, and (4) situation producing. Basically, nurse leadership practice relies upon the third and fourth levels of theories. The third level of theories is *predictive* theory, and the fourth level is *prescriptive* theory. These two levels enable the nurse-leader to formulate action hypotheses and to construct ways (or prescribe ways) in which one can create the environment or the series of events that will allow the prediction (action hypothesis) to come true. However, since a theory to be workable—to have reached its full maturity and have some chance at validity—must have evolved through the prior levels of development, the nurse-leader needs to have a working knowledge of all four levels of theories. In this way, nurse leadership action hypotheses (or predictive principles) have a much higher validity and reliability than those formulated in the limbo of the third and fourth levels, without reference to or cognizance of the prior two levels.

James Dickoff, Patricia James, and Ernestine Wiedenbach's classic article in *Nursing Research** provides the best source for a clear explanation of theory levels. Presented here is a highly simplified summary of the levels of theory in practice disciplines, as presented in their article.

Level I: Factor-isolating theories. Level I has two activities: (1) naming, or labeling, and (2) classifying, or categorizing.

Naming. The function of this basic stage is to allow an idea or object to be perceived and talked about or referred to. Once something is named, it is mentionable. One must isolate identifying aspects or factors to recognize that a thing is what it is and not something else, thus the title of this level: factor-isolating theories. Names may be assigned for a variety of reasons: (1) the order of discovery (such as the Caribbean hurricanes—Angela, Betty, Carol, Delphie); (2) the discoverer or inventor (such as Cushing's disease or Bowman's capsule); (3) by function (such as heart-lung machine or walkie-talkie); (4) similarity to other things that have previously been identified and named (such as kidney basin or kidney bean); and (5) by description (such as the black-backed three-toed woodpecker).

Classifying. The second activity in level I is classifying. Classifying is sorting, categorizing, or grouping things according to some commonalty. Classifying by commonality requires that the factors or attributes of an object, idea, or thing be *isolated.* The second activity is not possible without the first, that of perceiving and naming, having occurred. Categorizing requires one to identify

---

*Dickoff, J., James, P., and Wiedenbach, E.: Theory in a practice discipline. Part I. Practice oriented theory, Nurs. Res. **17**(5):415-35, 1968.

what something is and what it is not. Categories can be grouped just as single items can be grouped. Grouping or categorizing is possible because of some common denominator or unifying factor. Thus, a hierarchy of categories is formed. (*Acute inflammatory response* is a large category that contains subcategories such as *fever* or *local edema*.)

Level II: Factor-relating theories. Level II also contains two activities: (1) depicting, or describing, and (2) relating factors. This level of theory building depicts or describes how one, single, named and classified thing (factor) relates to another single, named and classified thing (factor), thus the title: factor-relating theories. For example, a description of the face requires communication of how the eyes sit in relation to the nose, mouth, ears, and forehead. This level of theory describes relationships to other factors. In other words, it is a "natural history" of any given subject. Any descriptive science, such as anatomy, is an example of factor-relating theory.

Level III: Situation-relating theories. Level III is concerned with causal relationships. It relates one situation to another in a way that allows for prediction. One of the essential ingredients of this level is causal-connecting statements that give a basis for prediction. Prediction is a statement of causal or consequential connections between two states of affairs, or two concepts. This level of theory reveals what conditions, circumstances, or behaviors (for example, the cost in time, energy, effort, pain) will promote or inhibit the occurrence of an event or consequence. Dickoff, James, and Wiedenbach consider this level of theory building to be of "incredible importance" to practice. Predictive principles, the format for this book, are in reality third-level theories. They are guides for developing realistic alternatives for nursing actions and are essential to the judgments and decisions of leadership. Simply stated, third-level theories tell you that if "A" occurs, "B" will occur. Third-level theories explain what promotes, speeds up, has a catalytic effect, slows down, inhibits, or prevents something from happening. Promoting or inhibiting theories indicate under what circumstances things will occur and with what speed and effort.

Level IV: Situation-producing theories. Level IV, the final level of theory building, comprises prescriptive theories; it is the level at which theories come to maturity. This level of theory indicates how one arranges the environment and circumstances so that the desired goal is achieved. Situation-producing theories have three aspects.

Goal. This aspect is the simple establishment of a goal. It is the primary act of any problem-solving organism. The nurse-leader is a goal-oriented human and has the behavior of helping others in goal identification and attainment.

Prescription. This aspect is a diagram or roadmap of the specific activities and directions that, when completed, will produce the results predicted in Level III (predictive theories) and achieve the desired goal. Prescriptions can be the actual directions for carrying out a plan necessary to achievement of a goal.

Survey list. The survey list contains the dimensions, knowledge, and other resources that might be helpful in structuring or completing the activity and provides the basis for judgments about alternatives in achieving the established goal.

Summary on theorizing

This book uses as its theoretical format predictive theories. Instructions in construction and use of predictive theories are provided for the nurse learning leadership. These instructions will show how second-level theories are used in constructing third-level theories. Problem solving is also one of the primary theoretical constructs of this book. Subsequent discussions will show how problem solving and decision making are, in essence, fourth-level theories. Problem solving produces the judgments and decisions necessary to select the series of actions that will achieve the desired result. In other words, the final act of problem solving is the selection of the series of actions or behaviors (prescriptions) that will produce the desired situation as predicted in the third level of theory building.

PREDICTIVE PRINCIPLES

Utilization of predictive principles in problem solving is based on a knowledge and understanding of theory levels and problem solving. Understanding the composition of predictive principle and the actions involved in using it is to acquire a *working definition,* or a definition that can be made operational. Real understanding of a definition comes when one has acquired the ability to use the definition in suitable activities. Some activities requiring the use of the definition of a predictive principle are identifying principles either in the literature or in use, constructing specific principles using the component parts (lower level theories) appropriately, and using principles in solving problems.

The following section begins with a working definition of a predictive principle and proceeds through the use of principles in solving a problem. This is designed to guide the nurse to an increased understanding of principles and enables the practitioner to use principles in activities that require leadership.

Definition

For use in this book, *a predictive principle is defined as a set of circumstances, conditions, or behaviors that produces a given, definable outcome.* A principle expresses relationships of conditions, circumstances, or behaviors to predictable consequences. A predictive theory is a nursing action hypothesis. Predictive principles differ from facts or concepts in that a fact or concept need only be valid, whereas a predictive principle, in addition to being valid, must predict outcomes. Principles are derived from authoritative sources or through scientific observation, experimentation, or compilation of data. Predictive principles are third-level theories.

The predictive relationships that exist between the circumstances, conditions, or behaviors and the predicted outcome or consequence of those circumstances, conditions, or behaviors can best be articulated by the use of an active verb or verb clause that is causal-connecting in a predictive way.

Predictive relationships may also be shown in two other ways:

1. "If-then"—if this happens, then this will happen.
2. Proportions—the greater this, the greater or less that.

Cause-and-effect relationships can be stated in future perfect ways because predictions are, in essence, an educated guess about what will happen in the future.

Below is an example of the definition in use. The example is fragmented into its component parts for illustrative purposes. In this book the word "valid" is used to mean empirically true; that is, that available evidence supports rather than refutes the predicted outcome.

EXAMPLE 1

Circumstances, conditions, or behaviors	Active verb	Given, definable outcome
A. Having knowledge pertinent to the current situation	assists the leader in making	valid judgments and decisions
B. The leader who has knowledge pertinent to the current situation	will be able to make	valid judgments and decisions
C. If the leader has knowledge pertinent to the situation	then he will be able to make	valid judgments and decisions
D. The greater his knowledge about the situation	the more likely the leader will be to make	valid judgments and decisions

Henceforth, for the purpose of brevity, the "circumstances, conditions, or behaviors" referred to in the above definition shall be known as the *CCB triad;* the "given, definable outcome" shall be known as the *predicted outcome* or the P.O.

Developing principles

The development of principles requires three stages of cognitive activity, which are the first three levels of theory building:

1. Identifying or accumulating facts and experiences or isolating and classifying factors (level 1 theory)
2. Depicting and describing factors or experience commonalities and relationships (This is a high-order conceptualization and is level 2 theory.)
3. Relating circumstances, conditions, and behaviors (situations) to consequences (level 3 theory)

Facts and theories can be fairly easily and rapidly identified and acquired through processes that enable and promote recall. Experiences (mental, emotional, and physical) allow for the further acquisition or retention of facts through the usage of learned material. Acquisition of facts could include such information as anatomy, physiology, or hospital or agency structure.

When facts begin to form a pattern and are applicable to several experiences, they become the second stage of cognitive activity, the formulation of concepts. For use in this book *a concept is a classification of experiences that have similar properties:* the recognition of commonalities for the purpose of useful classification. Concepts can be communicated to others. They can be converted into words or phrases which represent the ideas, objects, characteristics, or behaviors that are held together in groupings by the commonality. Concepts are the way people categorize experiences so that mental filing systems have organization. Concepts grow and enlarge as the number and variety of an individual's experiences increase. As examples, a compilation of facts, experiences, and observations concerning anatomy and physiology and the perception by the individual form the basis for the concept of pain. Facts related to hospital or agency structure serve as a basis for the formation of the concept of hierarchy. This activity is level II of theories.

The third stage of the development of principles is relating concepts to predict outcomes. This is a complex, but useful, thinking process because predictive principles show the relationship between concepts. *A predictive principle shows the relationship between the concept(s) drawn from the CCB triad and the concept(s) of the predicted outcome.* The concepts of *motivation* and *learning* will be used for illustrative purposes.

Motivation is a condition and is an example of a concept used as a CCB triad. Learning is an outcome and is an example of a concept used as the predicted outcome. Many discussions of the relationship motivation has to learning can be found in the literature. An observer of the learning process quickly recognizes that there is an inherent relationship between motivation and learning. The effect these two concepts have on each other can be expressed in a principle. The principle's components are separated in example 2.

EXAMPLE 2

CCB triad	Active verb	Predicted outcome
Being motivated	influences	learning

The above principle is simple and direct but is lacking in specificity and direction. The use of qualifiers gives principles increased usefulness. This is illustrated in the following way:

EXAMPLE 3

Having qualifiers	CCB triad	Active verb	Qualifiers	Predicted outcome
Being highly	motivated	increases	the rate of	learning

In the examples used thus far the CCB triad has always been on the left and the predicted outcome on the right. This is not necessary to the construction of a principle. To change the order of the concepts one need only change the orientation of the active verb phrase. The order of the concepts used in example 1 can be reversed as follows:

EXAMPLE 4

Predicted outcome	Active verb	CCB triad
Valid judgments and decisions	result more frequently when the leader has	knowledge pertinent to the current situation

The definition of a principle and the examples of principles used imply that the CCB triad with its qualifiers describes the environment, activities, knowledge, skills, or state of being necessary to make the predicted outcomes occur. The CCB triad is the concept subject matter and contains the necessary qualifying descriptions for the formation of prinicples. The CCB triad and its qualifiers can be positive or negative.

It is important to know what will produce, aid, ensure, or promote a desired outcome; however, it can be equally useful to know what will inhibit, prevent, or block a desired outcome. In the four examples given, the principles have been positive in nature. Negative CCB triads indicate what will not achieve the predicted outcome and, therefore, are used to formulate negative principles. These are inhibiting theories in level III of theory building. The following states the principle in example 1 negatively:

CCB triad	*Active verb*	*Predicted outcome*
Lack of knowledge pertinent to the current situation	inhibits the leader's ability to make	valid judgments and decisions

The active verb may also contain qualifiers. These are words that relate the CCB triad to the predicted outcome and may also tell who, how far, how much, how often, or what action takes place. Some words that indicate positive action are *facilitate, precipitate, aid, result in, determine, assist, influence, promote, ensure, contribute to, enhance,* and *enable.* Note that most of the action words suggested have limitations by definition. For instance, *facilitate* means to "make easy or less difficult," while *ensure* means to "make certain." The difference is important because the choice of the connecting action words helps to determine the validity of the principle. Some action words that indicate negative action are *inhibit, prevent, discourage, negate, invalidate, obviate, preclude, deter,* and *damage.* Active verbs, in addition to indicating the positive or negative direction of the activity, can, with qualifying phrases, indicate person. *Person* is the one who perpetrates the activity, for example, the nurse-leader, the learner, the patient, the ancillary worker, the student, or the group. It is not essential that person be indicated, but to do so promotes clarity and specificity. The following illustrates how different active verbs and persons alter the principle:

EXAMPLE 5

CCB triad	*Active verbs and person(s)*	*Predicted outcome*
Having knowledge pertinent to the current situation	(1) ensures that the leader makes (2) aids the group in making (3) promotes the making of (4) facilitates the making of (5) results in the group's making (6) helps the nurse-leader to make (7) enables the group to make	valid judgments and decisions

The above example indicates the variety of ways cause-and-effect relationships of a principle may be linked together. Choices are dependent upon the situation under consideration.

Clarity is achieved through accurate, concise statements of principles that are positive instead of negative, logical in their sequence, and contain connecting words and phrases that produce valid principles.

The Appendix contains detailed directions for the formulating of predictive principles. Nurses attempting to improve their leadership skills will find predictive principle formulation a valuable tool for acquiring and storing knowledge in a form useful for rapid decision making. Knowledge storage and retrieval in the form of facts makes no use of the practice implications. Predictive principles tie facts and experiences to practice consequences and thus are more useful to the nurse practitioners.

The Appendix also contains a few common construction errors made by the novice predictive principle formulator.

UTILIZATION OF PRINCIPLES IN SOLVING NURSING PROBLEMS

Organizing ideas and facts into predictive principles enables the nurse-leader to have a clear, categorized fund of knowledge for immediate use in nursing situations. However, the acquisition of a body of knowledge in the form of practical and usable predictions is only part of the problem facing the nurse who wishes to be a proficient leader. Predictive principles will have relevance only for the nurse-leader who judiciously applies them to identified problems. Predictive principles are guides for developing realistic alternatives of action. The use of predictive principles is a process that requires (1) identification of the real problem, (2) selection of the appropriate, valid, and relevant principle(s), (3) identification of alternatives for action sequential to the selected principle(s), (4) the ability to select one or more of the alternatives, and (5) the ability to prescribe the ways and means to actualize the alternative selected.

Initially this is a slow, laborious process, but through repeated application to various types of problems the process becomes a behavior habit. Habits of thinking beget habits of behavior. Habits are developed after thoughts or activities are repeated in the same pattern or way until the behaviors become customary. Habits are characterized by automaticity (without deliberation). Any skill, whether it is intellectual or manual, involves habits. (Even bed making was a slow process for the nurse at first.)

The mechanics of problem solving using predictive principles is a habit, not a reflex. Reflexes are inborn and inherent in the nervous system of the being; habits are learned. The answers to problems or possible alternatives of action do not materialize automatically; it is the *process* of arriving at the best possible alternatives that becomes the habit. When this process becomes habitual, the nurse-leader will automatically use the predictive principles approach to problem solving when faced with nursing problems. This means that each step in the process may lose its identity, become blurred, and may not be conscious; nevertheless, the process takes place. Arriving at this degree of skill requires consistent, repeated, conscious practice with positive reinforcement of successful use of the process.

Acquiring skill in problem solving must be reconciled with the needs of patients and the demands of agencies for ongoing nursing services. Nurses cannot cease activities or leave patients or team members in suspended animation and adjourn to the library to read about a topic and formulate principles. Real nursing problems, whether obvious or obscure, usually require some immediate action. Formulating and acquiring a list of principles, learning an organized methodology for problem solving, and enlarging the problem-solving tool chest and the critical thinking necessary to select the most effective nursing interventions are skills that must be learned initially in situations that permit time and freedom to err. One effective method is to allot a specified intervals when the involved personnel are relieved of nursing responsibilities and can work through the problem-solving process. Reality can be preserved by using problem situations observed in practice by the involved nurses.

Learning problem solving by using real problems in the class or conference room is a simulated problem-solving situation. Simulation, for the purpose of learning the role of problem solver, allows for practice of skills in a safe, non-threatening environment. Neither the nurse nor the patient or client can be severely damaged in a simulated environment. Mistakes in judgment, errors of commission or omission, are without deadly consequences. Yet, actual practice, an essential ingredient for learning any role, can be available. In the simulated learning situation, coaching can take place, complementary roles can be learned, the audience (classmates) can participate, and competence in decision making and other leadership skills can be acquired. However, though competence can be gained in simulated situations, only reality enactment of the role of leader-decision maker, can provide confidence in the nurse for that role.

After knowledge of principles and their use in solving nursing problems has been acquired, nurse-leaders can apply this knowledge to solve obvious nursing problems within the real situation with success and without disruption of necessary activities. The solving of complex or obscure problems frequently takes time and involves groups of people. The results of this group effort are (1) an increased awareness by the nursing group of nursing problems, (2) increased quality of nursing services to patients, (3) broadening and deepening of individual care giver's group nursing skill, and (4) utilization of each care giver's potential contribution to patient care.

Problem solving is a process. A process is an organization of many components, parts, other processes, and tasks to achieve an explicit purpose. The outcome of this combination of many factors is one unique episode, act, task, factor, thing, person, or process. The discussion of the processes of problem solving will be clearer if problems are divided into two categories—obvious and obscure. *Obvious* problems are problems open to view. In nursing they usually originate from procedures, schedules, timing, machinery, and work loads. *Obscure* problems are most frequently problems of behavior, communication, or interpersonal relations. Obscure problems are usually complicated by emotional overtones and loss of objectivity. In general, the more human interaction in an event or situation, the more difficult the identification and solution of the problem. Even overt problems may be difficult for the nurse-leader to identify because of strong distracting stimuli or inattention to or breakdown in the processes preliminary to identifying the problem.

The processes that produce clear and accurate problem identification are the same for both obvious and obscure problems; however, the steps for identifying obscure problems may be much more protracted than those used when identifying obvious problems.

Problems are continually being solved by every individual. It is impossible to go through life without some kind of successful problem solving, either conscious or unconscious, formal or informal. Problem solving is one of the most important elements of leadership in nursing. It becomes increasingly important that nurses enter the practice of nursing prepared to engage in an organized problem-solving process. One of the basic tenets of any group practice of nursing is that groups collectively are more productive, more efficient, and more effective than the sum of their individual members. The inclusion of other nursing care givers in problem solving whenever possible or appropriate ensures group commitment to the solution. This activity also improves esprit de corps, taps the abilities of each individual member, and gives the group the benefit of diverse thinking. The group process is slow at first but functions more rapidly as the group gains skill in problem solving together.

Problem solving has two aspects that nursing leaders must utilize (1) the tools or heuristics of problem solving and (2) the facets or phases of problem solving.

Problem-solving heuristics

Problem-solving heuristics are tools, techniques, or devices people use to solve problems. Whereas problem-solving facets or stages are aspects of problem solving (such as assessment, problem identification, and data gathering), problem-solving heuristics are the activities one uses in each facet to complete the tasks appropriate to that facet. For instance, some tools one might choose to use for assessment are looking, observing, questioning, or assuming. For problem identification, one might use the activities of guessing, assuming, supposing, analyzing, categorizing, synthesizing, or generalizing. Characteristically, every nurse-leader and every person being led has favorite problem-solving tools. Some people are impulsive and just leap in; some think the problem through from the beginning to the conclusion; and some work backward from a possible solution to the necessary supporting data. Some people tend to meditate or cogitate over problems; others let an idea incubate and come to a decision without conscious thought (sleep on it). The wider the range of problem-solving heuristics available to the nurse-leader, the more likely the leader will be to have at his disposal tools that will enable him to arrive at adequate decisions. No one heuristic or device is better than another; each has its use, depending upon the group, the leader, the problem, and the situation. Every nurse-leader must take inventory of his problem-solving tools, especially those he uses most frequently. He needs to watch and talk with others to find out what tools others use. By adding to his own tool chest and helping others add to theirs, he will expand his problem-solving skills and be more effective in facilitating the problem solving of others. Interaction Associates* has developed a list of problem-solving tools in common usage and has developed ways and means for facilitating the expansion of the tool repertoire for problem solvers.

Facets or phases of problem solving

Problem solving has four phases, facets, or stages. The term "facets" is used here because phases or stages communicate an order to the sequence of activities. Although listed here from problem identification to the judgment or decision, actually problem solving is seldom followed in that set sequence and order. The human mind tends to work backward and forward between aspects of problem solving until the completion or decision is reached. The development of data, alternatives, and other considerations throws light upon aspects of the problem previously developed, so that the whole changes; this flux is the process

---

*Strategy notebook, San Francisco, 1972, Interaction Associates.

nature of problem solving. Each facet of problem solving contains the tasks necessary for successful completion of that facet. No facet is static; each facet is dynamic, for information uncovered in one facet may alter the significance of the information uncovered in previous facets.

The following four facets of problem solving are designed for use in solving nursing problems. The steps of problem solving are in sequential form, and the tasks necessary to each facet are given. The following nursing problem is considered throughout to illustrate the use of this process.

PROBLEM: An aide on a nursing team failed to give oral care to the patients assigned to her.

Problem-solving facet I: Problem identification

Following are the tasks involved in problem identification:
1. Observe an event or situation.
2. Obtain relevant, valid, accurate, detailed descriptions from appropriate people or sources.
3. Write a description of the situation.
4. Discard irrelevant or questionable data.
5. Isolate the tentative problem and state it concisely.

TASK 1. *Observe an event or situation.* The first task of the problem identification facet is the recognition that a problem needs to be identified. It seems unnecessary to say that one must have a problem before the problem can be solved, but it is an important maxim. Problems, by definition, are a question or a perplexity. This means a process, activity, or normal progression of events has been interrupted, altered, or disturbed in some way. It means someone believes that the situation is not optimal or that expectations have not been met.

Nursing students are often given case histories of patients with directions to identify the nursing problems. In reality, these students are being asked to identify areas of nursing care necessary to the health of the patient. Specific problems cannot be identified without an event or situation that is not progressing normally or optimally. The following is a situation in which a team leader's normal expectations have not been met.

> While functioning as a leader of a team of nursing personnel on an acute medical care unit, the nurse notes that an aide on the team is not giving oral care to the patients assigned to her.

The team leader having observed this event or situation proceeds to task 2.

TASK 2. *Obtain relevant, valid, accurate, detailed descriptions from appropriate people or sources.* Accurate descriptions and observations are the forte of nursing; however, continued practice and study in this realm are necessary for maintaining and improving skill. Teaching observational skills to all nursing care givers will result in increasingly better nursing care. After one nurse-leader had repeatedly sensitized the ancillary personnel to accurate descriptions, an aide was asked in casual conversation if she had seen the director of nurses' new car. The aide answered that she had. The nurse-leader inquired about the color of the car. The aide responded that it was "blue on the side toward me." Although the aide's answer was facetious, this kind of cautious accuracy will increase the speed and validity of solving nursing problems through accurate and objective observations and reports.

Good results can be obtained by the nurse-leader if effective interviewing skills are exercised. Descriptions of situations collected from all individuals concerned can become confused and subjective if inappropriate questions are posed. Desired information can be obtained if the nurse-leader asks such questions as, "What happened?" "What preceded the event?" "What followed then?" "What else was going on while this was occurring?" "How did you feel about the incident?" Further data can be obtained by leading statements, "Tell me more about that," "Help me to understand the events." Sometimes simple listening postures and sounds are enough. Oh? Yes? and then. . .

Open-ended questions and statements such as these will assist the nurse-leader and those involved to separate feelings from facts and thus achieve objectivity and to formulate a more vivid description of the problem.

For example: the nurse-leader gathers the following descriptive information from appropriate sources.

1. There are twenty patients assigned to the nursing team on the given day; all but five are seriously ill.
2. Basic hygienic care to be administered to the twenty patients includes ten complete baths, five partial bed baths, five showers, and twenty beds to be changed; seven patients must be fed their meals.
3. One nurses' aide scheduled to work on the team failed to report to work because of illness. A replacement was not available.
4. Some team members had complained of overwork and expressed feelings of injustice.
5. The aide not giving oral care has been employed in this health agency for one month.

TASK 3. *Write a description of the situation.* The nurse-leader will find it helpful to take notes on the descriptions of the event as reported by all those concerned with the problem situation. Summarizing the descriptions in a short, concise, clear paragraph that contains all relevant material will aid the nurse-leader in clarifying the event. When events are in written form it is much easier to identify material that does not contribute to the description of the problem situation. Writing helps to crystalize thinking and is a valuable step in problem identification. A paragraph description of the problem situation is written below:

> An aide who has been employed one month is not giving oral care to patients assigned to her. Team members feel overworked with one unreplaced absent member. There are twenty patients, ten who need complete care and seven who need feeding.

TASK 4. *Discard irrelevant or questionable data.* Data that is irrelevant or of questionable use in identifying the problem may be of considerable use when gathering data for the solution of the problem. Superfluous material in the descriptive situation increases the confusion and difficulty of isolating the problem. This same data may be helpful at a different stage of problem solving. Below is the described situation with noncontributory material deleted.

> An aide who has been employed one month is not giving oral care to patients assigned to her.

TASK 5. *Isolate the tentative problem and state it concisely.* Problem identification is a dynamic not a static process. As information is gathered subsequent to the implementation of principles, it may become necessary to alter the original identified problem so that reality and accuracy are preserved. Identified problems should always be considered tentative or subject to change by the group or leader. When identified problems are labeled "tentative" there is greater willingness on the part of those participating in problem solving to change the identification of the problem. Groups and individuals can change the identified "tentative" problem with less embarrassment and with fewer feelings of inadequacy than they can a "definite" problem.

The temptation for the beginning problem solver is to put conclusions about why the aide is not giving oral care into the statement of the problem. Following are two possible erroneous statements of the above problem:

1. Aide not giving oral care because she resents her work load.
2. Aide inadequately oriented to ward routines and does not know she should give oral care.

Such guessing wastes time in idle speculation and leads to a search for substantiation of the hypothesis rather than selection of the appropriate principles and consequent activities necessary to the efficient and objective solution of the problem. Problems are easier to solve if stated as questions. Following is a concise statement of the problem:

How to alter the aide's behavior so that she gives oral care to patients.

Problem-solving facet II: Selection of appropriate principles

Following are the tasks involved in selecting the appropriate principles:
1. Determine topic(s) or area(s) of principles relevant to the subject.
2. Formulate the principles of the determined area or topic from authoritative sources appropriate to the tentative problem, or select appropriate list of principles from a cumulative file.
3. Select the specific principles applicable to the problem based on validity, relevance, and practicality.
4. List principles in the order they may be used most effectively.

Selection of appropriate principles is totally dependent upon the proper identification of the problem. Principles useful to the solution of the problem will be selected only if the correct problem has been identified.

TASK 1. *Determine topic(s) or area(s) of principles relevant to the subject.* Selection of the topic or subject of the principles is done by determining the subject area to which the problem relates. For example, if the nurse-leader concerned in this situation had identified the problem as "inadequate orientation," her principle area would have been "teaching-learning." Had she identified the problem as "resentment of work load," her principle area would have been "team spirit." However, the identification of the failure to carry out a job assignment properly clearly put the area of necessary principles as "delegation of authority."

TASK 2. *Formulate the principles of the determined area or topic from authoritative sources appropriate to the tentative problem, or select appropri-*

ate list of principles from a cumulative file. Nurse-leaders who utilize the principles method of problem solving accumulate large numbers of principles from which to draw. If the leader or group has no list of principles for the area selected, the principles will have to be compiled as discussed earlier in this chapter. However, if a list has been previously compiled, it should be examined for inclusiveness. If additional principles are needed, they must be formulated from authoritative sources and added to the list.

Nursing problems frequently require the utilization of principles from several subject areas. In the interest of simplicity, a problem has been chosen that can be satisfactorily solved using principles from one subject area. The following is a partial list of principles of delegation of authority from Chapter 4.

1. Written descriptions of policies, procedures, and/or guidelines by which an employee can handle situations when they occur promote ease of operation for the care giver and control of the authority delegated by the nurse-leader.
2. Member participation in the formulation of policies, job descriptions, and procedures increases member cooperation.
3. The philosophy and policies of a health agency determine the pattern of nursing care delivery system to be provided.
4. Guidelines, such as established channels, methods, and provisions for communication within an agency, enable the nurse-leader to delegate tasks and authority appropriately.
5. Clear lines of communication promote morale among organization members and enhance goal accomplishment.
6. A sufficient number of prepared personnel allows effective delegation of authority to meet organizational and patient needs.
7. Matching the abilities of the care givers to the jobs to be done increases work productivity and individual job satisfaction.
8. Assignments that have clearly defined standards and goals provide a basis for measurement of outcome.
9. Frequent comparison of actual performance with criteria determines the quality of care and the level of actual performance.

TASK 3. *Select the specific principles applicable to the problem based on validity, relevance, and practicality.* It is apparent that only selected principles within an area apply to a given problem. Some problems may require the use of only one or two principles for a solution to be reached; others may require many principles. The number of principles selected is dependent upon the nature of the problem.

After careful consideration the nurse-leader decides that the problem can be solved using principles 1, 4, 5, 7, 8, and 9. Principles 2 and 6 are not relevant.

The nurse-leader will evaluate each principle selected using the criteria of validity, relevance, and practicality. Principle 5 will be used as a model.

PRINCIPLE: *Clear lines of communication promote morale among organization members and enhance goal accomplishment.*

This principle is valid because if lines of communication are not clear or are not followed, mistrust develops rapidly in a group and morale decreases. For example, if the delegator has been unaware of each nurses' aide's activities, all team members might have been confronted for an explanation of the lack of good hygienic care. The use of this haphazard approach not only may offend the workers who are doing their jobs correctly but also may cause the team member involved to feel justified in offering retaliatory remarks such as, "You should have known that these patients were mine; you assigned them to me, so why didn't you come to me for an explanation?" The new employee may also feel insecure in her position and therefore take other means of self-defense; these usually involve "grapevine" activity that undermines the nurse as an effective leader.

The principle is relevant, for if the team leader knows to whom the responsibility for the patients involved is delegated, immediate personal contact can be established with that particular team member. The nurse-leader can then get immediate feedback about what is going on and why it is occurring. The principle is practical because it will work at the time and place needed within the natural limits of the situation.

TASK 4. *List principles in the order they may be most effectively used.* Principles show outcomes, and outcomes usually have a logical, necessary, desirable sequence. For example, the nurse-leader has channels-of-communication guidelines established by the agency; using those guidelines ensures that actions are within designated authority. Using established, designated lines of authority, the nurse-leader must take steps to ensure that the job descriptions, policies, and procedures include the assigned tasks and are available to each aide. The process of arranging principles in their logical order of use continues until all selected principles are arranged in an ordered sequence. The order in which the principles selected for the example problem can be most effectively used is as follows:

1. Guidelines such as established channels, methods, and opportunities for communication within an agency enable the nurse-leader to delegate responsibility appropriately (4).
2. Written descriptions of policies and procedures by which an employee can handle situations when they occur promote ease of operation for the team member and control of the authority delegated by the team leader (1).
3. Frequent comparison of actual performance with assignment determines the level of actual performance (9).
4. Clear lines of communication promote morale among organization members and enhance goal accomplishment (5).
5. Matching the abilities of the team members to the jobs to be done increases work productivity and individual job satisfaction (7).
6. Assignments that have clearly defined standards and goals provide a basis for measurement of outcome (8).

Flexibility in both the selection and order of application of principles is important. The result of an action dictated by a principle may necessitate the substitution of one or more subsequent principles. The nurse-leader familiar with all the important principles of a given area or topic finds flexibility easy to maintain.

Problem-solving facet III: Determining alternatives for action

Following are the tasks involved in determining alternatives for action:
1. Determine all alternative courses of action that are a natural consequence of each principle.
2. Determine who will select the course of action.
3. Select the courses of action(s) to be instigated and establish a serial order for implementation.

4. Evaluate selected alternatives for practicality. This requires determining if the proposed courses of action are:
   a. within the philosophy of the agency
   b. supported by the administration
   c. reasonable investments of time, energy, equipment, and money
   d. technologically current, yet within the abilities of the group
   e. assessed for safety and risk probability
   f. legally and morally acceptable to the nurse, group, and patient
   g. planned in conjunction with those who are most concerned with the problem (physician, patient's family, social services, occupational therapy, physical therapy, or rehabilitation personnel)

Facet III is a planning facet. Determining alternatives for action is a selective process in which one deliberates about the principles and the possible courses of action that arise from the principles, determines who must select the course of action, and attempts to establish the best *order* for implementing actions. Facet III is not the facet in which intervention behaviors occur; it is the facet in which plans, preparations, and decisions about intervention are made. Rapid judgments and decisions can be made by the nurse-leader, or discussions may be held with appropriate persons.

TASK 1. *Determine all alternative courses of action that are a natural consequence of each principle.* Since a "principle" is by definition a circumstance, condition, or behavior that produces a given definable outcome, activities are the natural extension of a principle. The activity consequence of a principle can take any number of forms depending upon the specific problem and ramifications of that problem. The consideration of a variety of alternative courses of action increases the probability of choosing a workable course of action. However, any activity considered must comply with the dictates of its antecedent principle.

In the example used here the following principle has been selected as the model: *clear lines of communication promote morale among organization members and enhance goal accomplishment.* This principle indicates that "clear lines of communication" is a condition necessary to maintenance of morale and the accomplishment of goals. Clear lines of communication can be achieved in a variety of ways depending upon the persons and the circumstances involved. Behaviors that lead to clear lines of communication are tailored to each individual problem or situation.

Following are some suggested alternatives for establishing clear lines of communication in the example situation:

1. Go immediately to the aide and ask for a conference.
2. Wait until there is a natural pause in her work and ask her to come for a conference.
3. Wait until her work is over for the morning and request a conference.
4. Go to the aide and tell her you wish to speak to her as soon as she can get free.
5. Give her a note asking her to come and see you as soon as possible.

The best way to establish clear lines of communication depends upon the persons involved and the circumstances. The nurse-leader must consider all alternatives and select the best for each situation.

TASK 2. *Determine who will select the course of action.* Selecting the course of action to be taken may not always be the responsibility of the nurse-leader. If the situation involves policy, procedure, patient safety or treatment, or cultural, religious, emotional, or interpersonal matters, the nurse may be compelled by policy, law, safety of the patient, or good judgment to involve other people in the selection of the appropriate course of action. In the example the *nurse-leader* will be the one to choose the alternatives to be used.

TASK 3. *Select the courses of action(s) to be instigated and establish a serial order for implementation.* As shown in task 1, each principle has one or more courses of action. In task 3 the nurse-leader must select the most effective actions from the list suggested in task 1. When the decision is made concerning the available alternative to be used, the order in which the courses of action are to be actualized must be determined. These activities are nursing action prescriptions and are in part level IV of theory building. The selected courses of action derived from the selected principles and arranged in the appropriate order for this situation would be as follows:

1. Seek out the aide in question.
2. Arrange a meeting in private with the aide.
3. Gather data that would determine the aide's:
   a. level of understanding of role
   b. ability to fulfill expectations
   c. reaction to the incident
   d. rationale for omission
4. Request the aide to give oral care to patients assigned to her (providing necessary assistance, teaching, and supervision).
5. Evaluate overall patient assignment to ensure continuing orientation and practice commensurate with experience and ability of all personnel.
6. Establish time for future conference.

TASK 4. *Evaluate selected alternatives for practicality.* Practicality is an important consideration. Prescribed action must be possible within a given framework at a specific time and place. "Common sense" or intuition is not sufficient. Social, physical, and biological science factors must be considered when testing principles for practicality. The practicality of any plan of action can be assessed through the use of the following criteria:

a. *Within the philosophy of the agency.* If the selected alternative is not within the philosophy of the agency, it is inappropriate for the nurse-leader to pursue that particular action. Policy is not the same as philosophy, but it reflects philosophy. For example, the philosophy of an agency may state that basic nursing care is to be provided or administered to every patient. Policy would then dictate that the one assigned to give care would follow through with the commitment.

b. *Supported by the administration.* Administration backing usually implies that policies and procedures have been formulated and that orientation has been provided. In the situation under question the nurses' aide, although a new employee, would have been exposed to appropriate procedure through in-service programs and supervision and would have had an opportunity to review the procedure manual at any time a need was felt.

c. *Reasonable investment of time, energy, equipment, and money.* Nurses have responsibilities for providing care to patients. Regardless of the agency involved, each patient is entitled to receive services according to his needs and according to the commitment of the agency to meet those needs.

The nurse-leader need not expend time and energy in determining if the service of oral hygiene should have been administered. All data support the need for this service. The next logical step is to investigate equipment. Were supplies available for the administration of oral hygiene? If not, why not? If so, why were they not used? The economic factor could play a part in this situation, depending on the philosophy of the institution. The health agency might expect each patient to provide his own equipment. If so, does the patient have supplies? When the institution provides equipment, supplies cannot be considered always available or unlimited in number. These are areas in which energy need be expended. Hopefully, the nurse-leader will have someone available to check nonnursing details; but in every case the responsibility for determining facts lies with the delegator of authority.

When emergencies arise, such as a reduction in the number of personnel, some goals are sacrificed and priorities among patients' needs are established. The authority figure will have the knowledge necessary to make judgments about the importance of oral hygiene in providing for the needs of an ill patient.

The leader of the nursing team will seek out the nurses' aide to find answers about why oral hygiene was not administered to the patients assigned to her.

d. *Technologically current, yet within the abilities of the group.* The field of technology includes scientific knowledge and mechanical and procedural skills. The investigator must know if the nurses' aide failed to administer oral hygienic care because of a lack of knowledge or skill. If lack of knowledge or skill is the reason, remedial steps are in order. The leader knows there has been a breakdown in initial orientation or continuing orientation.

There is a lag between current technology and worker's knowledge and abilities to implement technology. The field of oral hygiene has moved away from a simple gargle or a few strokes of a brush into a procedure that depends upon knowledge of anatomy and physiology, bacteriology, and dental hygiene. Patients have a right to the most technologically advanced care available, and nurses and employers need to keep abreast of advancements in order to provide the best care possible.

e. *Safety assessed and risk probability established.* In nursing, safety is always a primary consideration in selecting nursing interventions. Safety cannot be assumed for any act that has inherent risk. When selecting a realistic and usable alternative of action, one must consider what the gains and losses will be for the patient, his family, the nurse, and the hospital. Weighing risks and ascertaining the alternative that gives greatest benefit to the recipient of the action, with the least possibility of damage, can become quite complicated. The process can be compared to item pricing. If one goes out to buy a pair of shoes, one wishes to know how much quality and service can be obtained for how much money. All shoes cost something. The question becomes, "is the expected purchase worth the price?" There are times when the contemplated actions are simply not worth the risks involved, whether a health and safety risk or a social-interpersonal risk.

In the situation under consideration the team leader, in telling the aide about the omission of mouth care and asking for clarification, risks several things, among which are:

1. Offending or embarrassing the aide
2. Damaging rapport or relationships
3. Being placed in the vulnerable position of being asked why oral hygiene is important

If the omission is allowed to continue and nothing is done, the nurse-leader risks:

1. Reinforcing unacceptable behavior by silent consent
2. Allowing patient health, hygiene, and comfort to suffer
3. Criticism from team members who do give mouth care

The implementation of alternatives for each principle carries with it risks that must be evaluated. Actions and interventions will then be actualized in the full knowledge of the risks, and preparation can be made in anticipation of consequences.

f. *Legally and morally acceptable to the nurse, group, and patient.* Since nursing practice is governed by local, state, and federal regulations, most personnel are aware of basic laws concerning the practice of nursing. There are ample sources of reference if legal or moral issues become a question.

In the nursing situation posed the nurse-leader must be convinced that the nurses' aide did not omit oral hygienic care because of laziness. Serious moral and legal implications are presented if negligence is established. The supervisor of care realizes the possibilities of infection, malnutrition, and other problems that can occur as a result of omission of this important part of care.

g. *Planned in conjunction with those who are most concerned with the problem.* Many alternative solutions to problems involve others from numbers of disciplines, whether the problem be patient centered or organization oriented.

In the nursing situation under discussion the nurses' aide may need additional classes with the in-service education department, or more supervision from the nurse-leader, or she may need to participate in group discussion with members of the nursing team. All three alternatives may be desirable.

Problem-solving facet IV: Implementing intervention

Following are the tasks involved in implementing intervention:

1. Assume the responsibility for coordinating or implementing activities.
2. Determine what must be done to establish authority to implement the plan.
3. Establish time and place for follow-up, reassessment, and evaluation of activities.
4. Carry out plans.
5. Reassess, evaluate, follow-up, and revise plans according to data.

Facet IV is the action facet. All work prior to this phase has been in preparation. Facet IV is that phase in which the nurse-leader and nursing group have the responsibility for actualizing the philosophies, objectives, principles, and plans that have been previously determined. Facet IV complements the situation-producing theories (level IV) of theory building. They are prescriptive theories, which include the prescription, the implementation, and the evaluation of a nursing intervention.

Action requires not only implementing behaviors but also concurrent evaluation of the effectiveness of the action. Formalized reassessment is in part dependent upon data gathered during action. The following tasks of facet IV are the crux of the problem-solving process and are the proof of the validity of all the foregoing facets.

TASK 1. *Assume responsibility for coordinating or implementing activities.* A responsible leader is essential to the smooth implementation of alternatives. Often intervention activities occur over a period of several weeks. Patient problems are seldom solved quickly, and interdepartmental problems within an agency require continued effort, these activities require a leader who will be responsible for seeing that efforts are ongoing. This does not imply that the nurse-leader who assumes this responsibility will do all the work. It implies only that the leader will see that the planned activities are carried out.

The nurse-leader in the problem example is the organizational person most familiar with the situation and nearest to the level of operation. The responsibility for implementation and carry-through belongs at this level. Frequently nurse-leaders "pass the buck" for any number of reasons to those who might assume the responsibility for implementation. The head nurse or in-service education instructor is the most likely recipient of "buck passing." The nurse-leader must fully assume leadership responsibilities and act with the authority of the role. Any activities relevant to the patient care must be instigated and coordinated by the team leader.

TASK 2. *Determine what must be done to establish authority to implement the plan.* This task concerns authority. To carry out a selected alternative, the authority to implement an activity must be clearly established by going through the proper channels and lines of authority. Written memos are the best means of clearing channels or informing appropriate persons, regardless of the friendliness of relationships with line or staff people, other departments, or physicians. Conversations, both in person and on the telephone, that establish the authority to implement should be followed by a memo referring to the phone call or conversation and summarizing the content. These memos should be kept for future reference. Trust and good relationships are maintained through the use of good business practices. Good records of memos reinforce memory and provide a reference source. Reliance on memory alone is a shaky foundation for any relationship because it permits misunderstanding to occur without revealing to the participants that a misunderstanding exists, and, therefore, clarification is not possible. Memos reveal misunderstandings and allow the participants to clarify positions immediately. The memo also serves as a reminder of commitments or activities in progress. In this example, authority to act is invested with the position of team leader, and no other channels need be cleared.

TASK 3. *Establish time and place for follow-up, reassessment, and evaluation.* Establishing a time and place for follow-up and reassessment is important to ensure continuing awareness of and continuity in handling of the problem. Crisis situations invariably draw the strongest and most immediate response, and situations that have ceased to be crises are often delegated to places of less importance and are not followed through to completion. This practice increases the possibility that the same situation will again become a crisis. Planned follow-up establishes a system whereby further complications can be avoided and continued growth can be promoted.

Plans for follow-up and reassessment are most important when groups are involved in problem solving. Planned times for this important activity give the group a sense of continuity. It provides target dates and motivates individuals to think in realistic terms about what they can contribute to such a conference. This activity not only underlines the importance of the planned intervention but also allows the group to evaluate effectiveness and further plan other activities or even reassess the problem (see principle 6, problem-solving facet II, task 4, p. 21).

TASK 4. *Carry out plans.* The problem is identified, the principles selected, the alternatives established and chosen, authority clearly defined, and the implementation is under way. Nurse-leaders who are implementing plans and are wary of forgetting a part of the planned implementation may wish to make a list. This list, if made, should be kept small and brief.

When groups are involved, roles need to be clearly defined in the perpetration of a plan of action so that each person knows what every other person is doing. If all are to participate, *how* each will participate needs to be discussed so that guidelines for action are established and each person can fit within the framework.

In the situation under discussion the nurse-leader would find the appropriate aide, take her aside, and privately find out the information necessary. Basing his actions upon the findings of the interview, the leader would provide the necessary equipment, assistance, teaching, or supervision and arrange for the aide to give the oral care to the patients assigned to her. The team leader would arrange for further evaluation, assessment, and follow-up and evaluate the overall patient assignment.

TASK 5. *Reassess, evaluate, follow up, and revise plans according to data.* Task 5 occurs after the initial actions that deal with the immediate situation and is designed to determine if the problem has been adequately solved or if alterations in plans need to be made. Participation by all concerned is important to the success of this task. Retrospective as well as concurrent evaluation is necessary to the solution of any problem. The nurse-leader's evaluation, together with the aide's evaluation, will serve as a guide to determine the relevancy and effectiveness of all the problem-solving steps. Revision of plans may be necessary because of further developments, such as more trust and better communications, additional data, or the rapidity with which the aide learns. Procedure manuals or orientation programs may need review, or patient assignments may need more planning. This information may not become apparent until follow-up conferences in which all people concerned honestly attempt to evaluate the entire situation. From such conferences may come continuity and progress for the entire unit or a redefinition of the problem and subsequent problem-solving activities.

SUMMARY

This chapter provides the key hypotheses or theoretical constructs that form the premises upon which the rest of the book is based. Leadership is, in the final analysis, the ability to bring together many areas of knowledge and skill into a unified set of behaviors that facilitate the movement of individuals, families, groups, and communities toward a goal. This role enactment presumes knowledge and skill in role learning and role taking, analyzing and organizing life processes' components, theorizing, and problem solving and decision making. The ability to predict the consequences of a nursing act is one of the key cognitive processes of nursing problem solving. In other words, a predictive principle is a nursing action hypothesis and as such constitutes a limited nursing theory. The following five predictive principles summarize the theoretical framework of this book:

1. A clear operational definition of leadership facilitates role definition and role enactment.

2. Eclectic selection and synthesis of the many components of the processes of life enable utilization of these components in a unique, effective leadership act conducive to an established goal.

3. Conscious role learning, role taking, and role enactment and a large role repertoire facilitate more effective and efficient role adaptation and perception and response to leadership role needs.

4. Skill in theory identification, selection, and building enables identification of the level at which individuals and groups are operating and facilitates the use of appropriate behaviors that will complete the theoretical progression toward a desired end.

5. Skill in the use of problem-solving facets and heuristics promotes more effective and appropriate decisions and ease in helping others in participatory decision making.

BIBLIOGRAPHY

BOOKS

Bower, F. L.: The process of planning nursing care: a theoretical model, St. Louis, 1972, The C. V. Mosby Co.

Bruner, J. S., Goodnow, J. J., and Austin, G. A.: A study of thinking, New York, 1956, John Wiley & Sons, Inc.

Burton, W. H., Kimball, R. B., and Wing, R. L.: Education for effective thinking, New York, 1960, Appleton-Century-Crofts.

Gagne, R.: The conditions of learning, New York, 1965, Holt, Rinehart and Winston, Inc., pp. 31-61.

Hughes, B. C.: Men and their work, Glencoe, Ill., 1958, The Free Press, p. 120.

Interaction Associates: Strategy notebook, San Francisco, 1972, Interaction Associates, Inc.

Interaction Associates: Tools for change, ed. 2, San Francisco, 1971, Interaction Associates, Inc.

McDonald, F. J.: Educational psychology, Belmont, Calif., 1966, Wadsworth Publishing Co., Inc., pp. 48-67, 252, and 302.

Sarbin, T. R., and Allen, V. L.: Role theory. In Lindzey, G., and Aronson, E., editors: The handbook of social psychology, ed. 2, Reading, Mass., 1968, Addison-Wesley Publishing Co., Inc., vol. 1, pp. 488-567.

Smuts, J. C.: Holism and evolution, New York, 1926, The Macmillan Co.

Whitehead, A. N.: Process and reality, New York, 1929, The Macmillan Co.

PERIODICALS

Arndt, C., and Laeger, E.: Role strain in a diversified role set: the director of nursing service. Part I. Nurs. Res. 19:253-58, May-June, 1970; Part II. Sources of stress, Nurs. Res. 19:495-501, Nov.-Dec., 1970.

Dickoff, J., James, P., and Wiedenbach, E.: Theory in a practice discipline. Part I. Practice oriented theory, Nurs. Res. 17:415-35, Sept.-Oct., 1968.

Hall, J., O'Leary, V., and Williams, M.: The decision-making grid: a model of decision-making styles, California Management Rev. 7(2):43-54, 1964.

Schweer, M., and Gardella, F. A.: Planning, orienting, and preparing for a new kind of nurse leadership, Nurs. Outlook 18(5):42-46, 1970.

CHAPTER TWO

Principles of teaching and learning

ASSESSMENT

The learner's developmental stage, personal characteristics and prior experiences influence learning potential and dictate content.

The learner's sociocultural and religious group determines the nature, content, and acceptability of learnings.

The learner's prevalent life needs determine what he will learn.

FORMULATION OF OBJECTIVES

The more congruent and relevant goals are to life needs of the learner-client, the more likely the goals are to be achieved.

Participation of the learner in setting learning goals increases the number of learning activities meaningful and useful to the learner.

Realistic behavioral goal setting enables selection of appropriate and meaningful content.

Setting goals that specify the precise degree of attainment required provides the learner with guidelines that can be followed.

MOTIVATION AND REINFORCEMENT

An obvious relationship between learning activities and stated goals increases the motivational value of the activity.

Accomplishment of beginning objectives reinforces belief in ability and motivates to greater effort for greater accomplishment.

Closely monitoring the level and source of anxiety in the learner enables the teacher to adapt the learning plan to learner needs.

Teaching in times of crisis about how to handle the crisis increases the opportunity for reinforcement and retention of learned behaviors.

Rewards consistent with the value system of the learner such as recognition, praise, peer status, or valued gains are motivating and reinforcing influences and thus facilitate learning rate, amount of retention, and degree of behavior change.

Practice of learned activities in a variety of ways reinforces learned behaviors and promotes the ability to generalize and discriminate.

ESTABLISHING THE LEARNING ENVIRONMENT

A reciprocal relationship of trust and security facilitates teacher-learner communications and allows accurate assessment, learner participation in goal setting, and better utilization of resources.

Recognition of the effect environment has on learning enables the nurse-teacher to mobilize environmental factors for the reinforcement of content.

Making it explicit that accountability for learning rests with the learner enables the learner to meet his own learning needs and goals and enables the teacher to act as resource person, facilitator, validator, conferee, and consultant.

Verbal or written contracts with client-learners for attainment of specific learner needs enable the nurse-teacher to enact the teaching role more precisely and establish success criteria in collaboration with the learner.

Structure, limits, and feedback provide an environment that promote security and trust.

LEARNING ACTIVITIES

The more frames of reference (learning theories) the nurse-teacher is able to use, the more teaching strategies will be in his teaching repertoire.

Learning episodes that contain input, operations, and feedback increase retention and utility of learning.

The more teaching strategies and operations available to and usable by the nurse-teacher, the better able the nurse teacher will be to select a strategy based on learner and situational needs.

Utilization of problem-solving processes promotes continuity and ease of learning.

Content that flows from the familiar to the unfamiliar provides a point of reference and promotes efficient grasping of material.

EVALUATION

Objectives expressed as learner behaviors enable the teacher and learner to know the limits of expected outcomes and to evaluate in meaningful, specific terms.

All nurses function as teachers. Nurses teach patients, families, ancillary personnel, and each other. Teaching is inherent in the nurse role whether or not the nurse consciously cultivates and exhibits teacher behaviors. The formal classroom setting, where clearly delineated teacher-learner roles are established, is uncommon in staff nurse practice. Because of the nature of staff nursing the nurse-leader serves as teacher in a wide variety of common everyday activities. These activities range from role model in approaches and methods for solving nursing problems to preplanned teaching in small groups.

The staff nurse who assumes responsibility for assessing problems and for seeking ways to teach will be concerned with principles and methodology of the teaching-learning process. The problem facing all nurses is to develop structures and relationships in which learning can occur.

Vaccines are helpless to prevent diseases unless people use them; heart patients live longer if they learn how to cope with their disabilities; people with diabetes live fairly normal lives if they learn how to balance their body needs, food, and insulin; cancer can be diagnosed and treated early if people learn to watch for the signs and symptoms; contagion can be stopped when people learn how to intervene in the transmission system. The health status of any individual, family, community, or country is directly related to that individual's or group's (that person's or people's) ability to learn to prevent disease and to maintain health, to get well and stay well. Medical science is helpless against ignorance, and information is useless without changes in behaviors that translate the information into healthful activities.

Nurses are the single largest health worker force in the world. They teach health to people and in so doing prevent diseases, maintain health, facilitate coping, and enable individuals to learn to reestablish healthful living patterns. Several factors influence the teaching-learning process. These factors include (1) a need, problem, or dilemma that will motivate people to learn; (2) information that will enable people to make realistic decisions about behaviors; (3) support and direction that will enable people to alter behaviors to conform to decisions that have been made; and (4) reinforcement, which will ensure the continuation of changes in behavior.

Teaching is often considered to be primarily a process of giving information to others; however, information alone will not enable the learner to change his behavior. As T. S. Eliot wrote in "The Hollow Men,"

Between the idea
And the reality
Between the motion
And the act
Falls the Shadow.

The nurse-leader who teaches individuals and groups must ensure that applicable information is available and, additionally, must help the learner translate that information into behaviors so that no "shadow" falls between the idea and the behavior.

A teacher is a catalyst in that he can bring knowledge and learner together and stimulate a reaction. The teacher can engage in activity that either facilitates or inhibits the reaction; he can function in ways that make the reaction either transient or more stable. Teaching causes learning to take place. Learning is the acquisition of knowledge with subsequent changes in the behavior of the learner. Behavior, as used here, means anything a person does in response to an internal or external stimulus. This response can take the form of overt physical activity, emotions, or mental processes. Teaching and learning are inseparably linked in a cause-and-effect relationship and are consequently treated here as a single topic.

Teachers work with feelings just as often as with information, for teaching is done with human beings. It is a popular misconception that if the teacher is dealing with feelings, the activity is not teaching but psychotherapy. There is conflict and disagreement among authorities about the similarities and differences between psychotherapy and teaching. Teachers are anxious not to blunder into areas that should be handled by a skilled therapist and are eager to establish some way to discriminate between the two. Basically, both psychiatric therapy and teaching have as their purpose behavioral changes, and this is what generates much of the confusion. In both teaching and therapy the client or the learner must rearrange relationships between himself and other people, himself and a task, or himself and his environment. One of the key differences between the person needing therapy and the person needing teaching is the degree to which society has difficulty with the person. The person who needs psychotherapy is perceived either by himself or by others as behaving in a socially unacceptable manner. The person who needs teaching may not be using himself to his fullest potential, but he is not ostracized by society. The difference is essentially a matter of degree.

Nurses must exercise considerable judgment in determining the differences between teaching and psychotherapy. There are few definite rules, but there are some guidelines that will help the nurse-teacher to determine if the teaching role is appropriate. Following are some of these guidelines:

1. Does the learner have the mental and physical potential to learn (can he alter his present behavior to the desired behavior)?
2. Does the learner have a behavioral or thought disorder?
3. Can changes in behavior be brought about by:

   a. increased self-awareness and sensitivity to others?
   b. additional information?
   c. additional physical or cognitive skills?
   d. additional choices or alternatives?
   e. change in habit patterns?
   f. encouragement, reinforcement, or evaluative feedback?
The following example illustrates the use of the above criteria:

> Mr. Nesbit, a 38-year-old man, was suffering his first episode of duodenal ulcers. The nurse making the initial hospital admission contact with Mr. Nesbit asked him if he had any idea why he had ulcers. Mr. Nesbit replied that he thought he knew. He stated that there were times when he could feel his "stomach tighten up and the acid just pour out." When the nurse reported this to the team, the group asked, "Why not teach this man a different way to handle his feelings so that he need not jeopardize his health?" The nurse-leader replied, "I can't do that, I'm not a psychiatrist!"

The group decided to apply the criteria to determine if they could teach Mr. Nesbit and thus change his behavior response to feelings.

The following is the use of the criteria and the group's findings. No effort is made to discuss clinical content. The focus of the discussion is on the methodolgy of the utilization of the above criteria for the preparation of patient teaching plans.

Criteria	Group conclusions
1. Has the mental and physical potential to learn.	Mr. Nesbit is of normal intelligence, has no physical handicaps, and has held a stable job for many years.
2. Does not have a behavior or thought disorder.	The patient has socially acceptable behavior, can carry through in ordinary conversation, and makes appropriate responses to interview questions.
3. Changes in behavior can be brought about by:	
a. Increased self-awareness and sensitivity to others.	Mr. Nesbit indicated an honest and well-developed sense of self-awareness as early as the first contact.
b. Additional information.	Additional information about stress, ulcers, and his behavior was available that would provide further data upon which the patient could base changes of behavior.
c. Additional physical or mental skills.	Earlier awareness of rising stress would enable him to perceive impending situations that would elicit gastric responses.
d. Additional choices or alternatives.	Mr. Nesbit could participate with the nurse-teacher in exploring helpful ways to deal with stressful situations.
e. A change in habit patterns.	Once new ways of handling stress are identified and tried, successful ones can be developed into new habits.
f. Encouragement, reinforcement, or evaluative feedback.	Close and honest working relationships with Mr. Nesbit can provide the nursing staff with opportunities to participate in identifying and reinforcing successful ways of handling stress. Reduced acid flow will be reinforcing.

When the above discussion was completed, the team decided to work with Mr. Nesbit and teach him a more healthful way to handle stress. The nurse talked extensively with the patient and discovered that with some direction he could identify some recent, very consistent sources of stress. The nurse supplied information about the pathophysiology of duodenal ulcers, and together Mr. Nesbit and the nurse worked out several alternative ways of dealing with the stress at the time it occurred. His hospital stay was of sufficient length to allow him several opportunities to cope with stressful situations successfully. The nursing team collaborated to reinforce his changing behavior.

ASSESSMENT

Assessment is determining the present status of the individual; goal setting is establishing the changes that are necessary; teaching is facilitating changes; and evaluation is assessing what changes occurred and whether they were the desired changes.

Assessment is the first step in the teaching process and is necessary to establish need, content, and method. Even when incidental teaching occurs, quick assessments are made by the nurse-leader. Often these are so natural they are engaged in without planning or conscious thought. Some of these easy and obvious assessments are the general health status of the learner, his age, general alertness, and any of his more obvious characteristics.

Planned change requires detailed and methodical assessment of the learner and those things that influence his learning. Assessment is not something that ends before teaching begins; it continues throughout the teaching process. Information gathered during all phases of teaching adds to the teacher's total knowledge of what the learner brings to the teaching-learning situation, and this knowledge contributes to better teaching.

The effective teacher gathers information from all available and appropriate sources. The patient, family members, friends, others members of the nursing and health teams, charts, observations, and other agencies contribute to the total data about the learner. The principles elaborated in this section are designed to help the nurse-leader assess the learner so that content and methodology have meaning and are useful.

PRINCIPLE: *The learner's developmental stage, personal characteristics, and prior experiences influence learning potential and dictate content.*

The age and central stage of development of the learner will determine how he interprets what he hears, sees, and experiences.

The age level is an indication of "normal" growth and maturation. The average child grows at a given rate and develops physical and mental skills at certain mean ages. With knowledge of normal growth and maturation the teacher will know at approximately which ages muscular coordination is developed, abstract thinking is developed, and when physical decline will begin to occur.

Erikson's stages of development are briefly outlined below. Only the positive senses are listed. The negative senses, which Erikson calls the "dynamic counterpart," are omitted for brevity. The development of these "senses" is a problem or task facing each individual.*

---

*For a full discussion of the stages of development see Erikson, E. H.: Childhood and society, ed. 2, New York, 1963, W. W. Norton & Co., Inc., pp. 247-273.

1. Sense of trust (first year)—satisfying experiences or finding biologic and emotional needs taken care of consistently in appropriate ways without pain or harm
2. Sense of autonomy (12 months to 3 or 4 years)—asserting and concluding that he is an individual with a choice and responsibility
3. Sense of initiative (4 to 6 years)—finding out what he can do; period of vigorous learning and intrusion into other people's worlds by physical attack, incessant questioning, and locomotion
4. Sense of industry and accomplishment (6 to 12 years)—engagement in real, worthwhile, socially useful tasks that can be completed correctly and well
5. Sense of identity (early adolescence, 12 to 15 years)—clarification of who he is, what his role in the world will be, and to what group or groups he belongs; whether he is independent or dependent, adult or child
6. Sense of intimacy (middle to late adolescence, 15 to 20 years)—friendship and companionship; need for warm, close bonds with others, even a need for an inner feeling of fusion with others
7. Sense of generativity (adulthood)—interest in producing and caring for one's own children
8. Sense of integrity (maturity)—healthy integrated personality that accepts his life, limitations, people, group, and time period; recognition and acceptance of limitations and potentialities

These categories are presented briefly and incompletely. The ages given are approximate ages of focus for each task. No task is mutually exclusive of other tasks, and most of them overlap and are repeated at subsequent stages of development.

The nurse-leader who can recognize the developmental level and central tasks of the learner can use this knowledge effectively in teaching. For example, the child who has not developed a concept of time cannot be taught about "tomorrow," for time has no meaning or reference point. The 6- to 10-year-old child can best be taught by utilizing his sense of industry and accomplishment, and the adolescent can be taught by using his sense of identity and independence from adult domination.

The use of central tasks of development in teaching patients can be seen in the following situation:

> Carolyn, a 16-year-old girl, was admitted to the orthopedic ward with a fractured femur and was placed in balanced traction. She was 30 pounds overweight and was placed on a 1,000 calorie diet. Maintenance of the diet quickly became a power struggle between Carolyn and the nursing and dietary staffs. The physician ordered dietary teaching for Carolyn, which was given by the hospital dietitian using didactic methods.
>
> High school friends participated in the power struggle by smuggling in favorite candies; parents became caught up in the cross fire between pampering a loved child and cooperating with the prescribed regimen. One day the team leader said, "Carolyn, does food really mean that much to you?" Carolyn replied, "Not really, but I don't like to be *made* to do anything. I'm old enough to eat what I please."

The nurse assessed Carolyn's present task of development as the need for identity and independence from adult domination. This developmental task was then used by the nurse to foster personal growth. The nurse obtained the physician's cooperation, and the diet order was changed to a "regular select." The nurse then acted upon the knowledge that the adolescent needs to plan his own life and course of action in collaboration with others but with some degree of independence.

The teacher used Carolyn's additional need for intimacy with the concomitant adolescent preoccupation with appearance and attraction of the opposite sex to interest her in personal hygiene and grooming. Dietary facts and information were supplied in the form of booklets and pamphlets. Carolyn was soon asking for explanations about food values, calories, fats, protein, and carbohydrates. A high school friend brought her a home economics book, and Carolyn requested the dietitian to come back so questions could be answered. By the time Carolyn returned to school, she had lost the 30 pounds and was helping her mother lose weight by planning the family meals. The nurse's skilled use of the central tasks of development of the middle teens enabled the accomplishment of the desired health goal for Carolyn.

Personal characteristics, such as intelligence, curiosity, perseverance, ways of handling stress, and adaptability, help to determine the content and method of teaching. Often a learner's inability to speak English, or health problems, such as blindness or deafness, mask intelligence or obscure other personal characteristics. These factors should be carefully considered when assessing the learner.

The nurse-teacher can make some personal characteristic assessments by observing the learner's ability to solve small problems and cope with minor life situations. Entering into ordinary discourse with people can give the nurse further clues about their intelligence and level of curiosity. The nurse can observe (1) the kind of questions that are asked; (2) the frequency with which the same question is repeated; (3) the rapidity with which simple instructions and routines are grasped; and (4) the difficulty or ease with which new ideas and ways are adapted. These observations help the nurse build a picture of the learner's personal characteristics and assist with the adoption of content useful to the learner.

Prior experiences influence present responses by providing the conditioning and context for understanding the meaning of educational stimuli. Concepts are learned by building ideas, facts, knowledge, and antecedent concepts, one upon the other, pyramiding them into an interrelated whole.

Everyone has antecedent knowledge and concepts upon which to build new knowledge. The nurse cannot assess all prior experiences of learners but can evaluate selected prior experiences. Education, family, constellation, experiences with teachers and health personnel, hobbies, interest areas, or occupation provide reference points, context, and antecedent knowledge for learning. This information allows the nurse-teacher to start where the learner is and to relate new material to familiar material in meaningful ways.

PRINCIPLE: *The learner's sociocultural and religious group determines the nature, content, and acceptability of learnings.*

The learner's sociocultural and religious group usually determines his value system. The value system dictates what is right and wrong, moral and immoral, fair or unfair, honest or dishonest, desirable or detestable. A value system influences ideas and feelings about others and provides guides to behaviors.

Teaching and learning objectives consistent with the learner's value system are realistic and achievable; the value system itself can be used as a motivation factor. Objectives in conflict with the learner's values are unrealistic and almost impossible to achieve without first changing the values.

An example of the influence of values derived from cultural groups can be seen in the following:

> Alfonso is a 22-year-old Mexican-American with diabetes. Alfonso resisted all health teaching, regardless of methodology, until he saw another diabetic, aged 40, with a below-the-knee amputation as a result of gangrene. The knowledge that a loss of limb could be a consequence of uncontrolled diabetes and inattention to special foot care shocked Alfonso and threatened his "macho" (self-concept of manliness). He became interested in preserving his feet and legs and learned rapidly about all aspects of diabetes. He also helped the nurse to understand the importance of the "extended family" in the Mexican-American culture so that more valuable and realistic teaching could include reference to the "extended family."

Knowledge of and respect for the learner's value system will be a major determinant in the teacher's success or failure and may influence the learner's future relationship with health care personnel. Values govern both the learner's and the teacher's behavior; interpretations of and judgments about other people's behavior are made within the framework of each person's value system. The nurse-teacher must not only be cognizant of the learner's sociocultural or religious values but also must have insight and self-knowledge.

PREDICTIVE PRINCIPLE: *The learner's prevalent life needs determine what he will learn.*

The learner, as does any other organism, responds to the strongest stimulus. A strong need is a strong stimulus, and the teacher must identify early the most urgent need, for until this need is met, little else will be learned. The needs of the learner determine what he will see and hear and the interpretation he will place on sensory input. A patient who had just had an electrocardiogram and who was anxious over the results was asked by the team leader, who was making patient rounds, if he had been up yet that morning. The patient replied, "Why, what's the matter, is something wrong with my EKG?" Another patient, responding to a different need, might reply, "No, not yet, I wake up slowly, and I haven't had any coffee yet."

A strong stimulus can create a need and facilitate learning or can interfere or distract the learner so that the stimulus becomes an inhibitor. A patient who is concerned about an errant husband or a sick child may not be able to learn about prenatal diets because of the more pressing worry.

Selective hearing, need, and readiness become problems to the teacher only if the teacher has not assessed the most pressing and current need of the learner collaboratively with the learner. Frequently what the learner wishes and is ready to learn is more important and achievable than what the nurse wishes and is ready to teach. Developing common goals may require a synthesis of teacher and learner goals.

FORMULATION OF OBJECTIVES

An objective is a destination, goal, or an expected or desired outcome. An objective defines where ones wishes to go and what one wishes to accomplish. It tells what the learner will be able to write, recite, construct, identify, differentiate, contrast, solve, compare, discriminate, judge, do, and so on. Objectives tell the teacher what is to be taught and the learner what is to be learned, and they enable both to determine the extent of accomplishment.

Objectives cannot be assumed, for such assumptions lead to conflict of purpose and misunderstandings and defy evaluation. Objectives need to be clearly and concisely stated so they can be understood, accepted, and used. Vague objectives, couched in erudite but trite jargon, are useless to most teaching-learning participants. Simple, direct, and explicit sentences that spell out in common language the desired outcomes enable the teacher and learner to select content, methods, materials, and activities that are appropriate and can promote goal accomplishment.

PRINCIPLE: *Participation of the learner in setting learning goals increases the number of learning activities meaningful and useful to the learner.*

PREDICTIVE PRINCIPLE: *The more congruent and relevant goals are to life-needs of the learner-client, the more likely the goals are to be achieved.*

Setting goals with the learner helps to keep them realistic and meaningful. Participation of the learner in goal setting enables goals to be set that are within the framework and context of his life and needs and ensures that established objectives are goals to which he is committed.

Learners have information, insights, awareness, and cognizance of problems pertaining to their own lives and needs; the teacher has specialized knowledge, skills, experiences, insights, perspectives, and often an objectivity that the learner does not possess. Working together, teacher and learner can set goals best suited for specific needs.

PRINCIPLE: *Realistic behavioral goal setting enables selection of appropriate and meaningful content.*

PREDICTIVE PRINCIPLE: *Setting goals that specify the precise degree of attainment required provides the learner with guidelines that can be followed.*

Inevitably, content is dictated by goals. Specific behavioral objectives enable the teacher to determine what content is realistic and relative to the attainment of each goal. The teacher need only answer the question, "What does the student need to learn in order to behave in the described manner?" to select the specific content necessary to goal achievement. This is seen in the following example:

GOAL: To be able prior to discharge to change the dressing on your leg using aseptic technique.

Attainment of this goal requires a knowledge of the concepts of asepsis from which theories of asepsis are comprised, a knowledge of selected bacteriologic facts, and principles formulated on the basis of those facts. Achievement of the above goal requires a knowledge of the dangers or risks involved and an ability to make valid judgments and discriminations when applying a sterile dressing in a variety of circumstances. Finally, attainment of that goal requires the enactment of specific behaviors.

The actual content selected to be taught or included is influenced by the assessment of the learner—his previous experience, his basic bacteriologic knowledge, and his particular needs. When the goal is *the ability to change a dressing using aseptic technique,* two hours are not spent discussing the pharmacologic properties and physiologic action of penicillin, even though there is a tenuous relationship of topics. In other words, specific goals help to decrease tangential and noncontributory activities.

Without specific, realistic goals, content selection becomes arbitrary and is frequently motivated more by what the nurse-teacher is comfortable in teaching than by what the learner needs to know. Therefore realistic, specific, behavioral goal setting gives structure to learning situations, which decreases the frustration and lowers the anxiety of both teacher and learner by enabling the learner to understand how content will be useful to him.

MOTIVATION AND REINFORCEMENT

Theorists differ in basic assumptions about the role of motivation and reinforcement in learning. In this discussion no attempt is made to explain or reconcile differences among learning theorists, but an attempt is made to choose those theories or aspects of theories that will be most helpful to the staff nurse during her everyday teaching responsibilities.

Motivation can be intrinsic or extrinsic. Intrinsic motivation is the impetus, incentive, or driving power within an individual that propels him into action. The teacher who can capitalize on an individual's motivation can concentrate on the activities of being mentor, guide, validator, supervisor, enabler, supporter, reinforcer, and evaluator. Extrinsic motivation is provided by the teacher or other external factors that influence the learner's desire to learn. These factors can be identified and manipulated to maximally develop and directionally influence learner motivation.

The nurse-teacher will discover that motivation may be influenced by personal and individual circumstances but that intrinsic motivation is the most important of the two types of motivation. Some motivating factors are common to most individuals and groups. This section relates to the common principles of motivation and learning and is primarily concerned with intrinsic motivation.

PRINCIPLE: *An obvious relationship between learning activities and stated goals increases the motivational value of the activity.*

The more reasonable and meaningful the activities appear to be to the learner, the more effort he will invest in their accomplishment. For example, the patient or aide learning about changing dressings using aseptic techniques may balk at learning the physical principles governing the capillary action of fluids until he sees the influence of those principles on the transportation of microorganisms by moisture.

The nurse-teacher can demonstrate relationships between necessary knowledge antecedents, content, and objectives by planning overall teaching content with the learner in a graphic way. To the uninitiated learner, knowledge basic or preliminary to goal accomplishment may appear to have little relevance to the goal. Content and activity plans, either written or carefully described so that relationships between necessary learning activities and accomplishment of goals will be conspicuous to the learner, can stimulate motivation.

PRINCIPLE: *Accomplishment of beginning objectives reinforces belief in ability and motivates to greater effort for greater accomplishment.*

Probably nothing is quite so motivating as success. Success is a lessening of anxiety or tension because a goal has been achieved. It is a moment of accomplishment when confidence grins a little and takes a deep breath. The next task is then begun with confidence reaffirmed and reinforced. Anxiety about failure is somewhat relieved, and fear of falling short of an established goal is decreased.

Success early in the learning process is necessary even to those who appear most confident. The nurse-teacher who sets a few small but challenging goals that can be met early in the learning process ensures greater motivation and effort for the larger learning tasks. Success can be planned by structuring learning situations with a high probability of success. The reinforcement of having succeeded, even in a small learning task, can be highly stimulating to the student and can motivate him to greater effort. Success early in learning will promote greater tolerance of failure.

PREDICTIVE PRINCIPLE: *Closely monitoring the level and source of anxiety in the learner enables the teacher to adapt the learning plan to learner needs.*

PREDICTIVE PRINCIPLE: *Teaching in times of crisis about how to handle the crisis increases the opportunity for reinforcement and retention of learned behaviors.*

People do not learn until an obstacle, obstruction, puzzle, dilemma, or interruption of some kind is encountered. Under ordinary circumstances this interruption creates a state of mild anxiety, and resources are mobilized to overcome, solve, or bridge the problem. At this stage the learner is highly motivated to learn things that will contribute to his ability to solve the problem or achieve his goal. Statements such as, "I function more efficiently under pressure," refer to the level of anxiety described above.

When the pressure is increased, anxiety increases and diminishing returns are realized. The learner's activities are no longer goal oriented and tend to function as a pressure release valve without actually contributing to solving the problem itself. Activities such as telling everyone how overworked one is, making elaborate preparations for work, and making several trips gathering books or equipment when one trip would suffice are all clues to the teacher that learner anxiety has increased.

Mild anxiety is the natural state of the human organism. Dynamic tension is the mechanism by which homeostatic balance is maintained. The healthy state is not a tension-free state; it is a state of tension balance. Anxiety is a pivotal learning force. Without some level of anxiety, no learning takes place. Anxiety is always a result of encountering a problem. Sometimes the anxiety is so mild it is not readily observable, or it may not be within the learner's level of aware-ness. Encountering a problem, or if you prefer, recognizing a goal, is always accompanied by an internal "toning up," a sharpening of wits, an increase of alertness that is called anxiety. McDonald* calls this anxiety state an "intra-personal energy change." Anxiety thus becomes the precursor to motivation. McDonald characterizes motivation as a condition necessary for learning but not sufficient to make learning occur. He defines motivation as having three char-acteristics: (1) intrapersonal energy change, (2) affective arousal, and (3) antic-ipatory goal reaction. The "intrapersonal energy change" may be caused by autonomic response mechanisms (as with fear) or basic life support needs. Most of the time the exact nature of the causal sequence of the energy change is unknown. The "affective arousal" is a feeling state or emotion. This state may not be in awareness or it may be a highly charged, intense emotion and well within the level of awareness. The "anticipatory goal reaction" is the purposeful-ness of motivation. Motivation is goal oriented, for it is through movement toward the goal that anxiety is reduced and satisfaction or pleasure is achieved. The con-sequence is that goal achievement returns the arousal state to normal and reduces the energy change to its prior level.

Generally speaking, the higher the anxiety, the more specific and focused the learner's attention, so that learning goals unrelated to the anxiety are not achieved. Learner attention becomes highly focused on the stimulus causing the anxiety. Teacher activities either begin to center around reducing the anxiety, strengthening coping mechanisms, or around teaching coping behaviors directly related to the source of the anxiety. Crisis, a state of very high anxiety and acute problems, provides a fertile field for learning. The person in crisis needs solutions so desperately that he is very receptive to cues and models, information guidance, and so on. The nurse-leader who takes the person in crisis through the activities necessary to resolve the crisis is capitalizing on prime learning time. The learner uses a real situation to learn behaviors that are immediately useful and have instant reinforcement.

Anxiety is one of the most delicately balanced factors influencing motivation. Perception of anxiety, accurate assessment of the levels of anxiety, and responses designed to control anxiety can mean the success or failure of any teaching endeavor.

PRINCIPLE: *Rewards consistent with the value system of the learner such as recognition, praise, peer status, or valued gains are motivating and reinforc-ing influences and thus facilitate learning rate, amount of retention, and degree of behavior change.*

Reinforcement of desired behaviors is the most influential factor contributing to the retention of learning. Reinforcement takes many forms and assumes many meanings depending upon the reinforcing stimuli and the learner's value system.

Recognition of a successful experience is a prompt reinforcement. Success

*McDonald, F. J.: Educational psychology, Belmont, Calif., 1966, Wadsworth Publishing Co., pp. 111-113.

is probably the greatest reinforcer. The nurse-teacher can promote the reinforcing value of success by preparing the learner to recognize the characteristics of a successful experience. Behavioral objectives that are spelled out enable the learner to identify what successful behaviors are and to recognize his own success immediately.

Reward and punishment reinforcement is helpful, depending upon the form it takes. Reward tends to be more successful than punishment. Rewards can be something tangible received for desired behaviors or positive feedback that causes good feelings. For instance, the relief of anxiety, as discussed above, can be an important positive reinforcer.

Recognition by others can be highly reinforcing. Success recognized and appreciated by a meaningful individual or group and mentioned to other people important to the learner acts as a strong reinforcer in the learning experience.

For employees, rewards may take the form of statements in efficiency reports, letters to the employer or supervisor, commendations made to committees on promotions, and written memos to people in a position to give employment rewards such as salary raises, promotions, bonuses, and educational leaves. Copies of all such commendations should be sent to the employee.

Reinforcement therapy is being conducted currently for both selected psychiatric and pediatric patients. This reinforcing method uses rewards of valued objects, tokens that can be exchanged for privileges, favored foods, candy, or other desired objects as tangible rewards that can reinforce desired behaviors effectively. There must be careful selection of candidates for the controlled use of this teaching technique, for if used inappropriately, it can become a way to obtain a desired object rather than a way to learn successfully.

Status rewards can be very important to learners. "Face," family pride, superior achievement, special mention, or public acclaim can fit into a value system and fulfill a need that can be more reinforcing than any tangible form of reward.

Punishment is an often-used negative reinforcer, but it has limited effectiveness in the teaching-learning process. Punishment of patients usually takes the form of reprimands, deprivation of privileges, exhibition of angry behavior by authority figures, ridicule, or sarcasm. Punitive statements such as, "I'm not speaking to you today; I heard how bad you were last night," or "That was a stupid thing to do; what in the world made you do that?" do not contribute to the motivation of the learner and probably only serve some ego need of the nurse-teacher. Punitive measures may cause the learner to avoid the teacher and withdraw from learning situations. Fear of punishment or failure can cause learners not to try. This does not imply that failure should be ignored, nor can the teacher positively reinforce *nonlearning,* for that would negate *positive* reinforcement of *learning.* The teacher can make an evaluative statement about whether the objective has been accomplished and/or can help the learner learn to evaluate his own progress.

The optimal use of the reinforcements most meaningful to each individual requires the nurse-teacher to utilize the reinforcement judged effective for each person or group in each separate learning experience. The closer the reinforcement follows the successful learning experience, the more valuable the reinforcement for both motivation and retention. Continued reinforcement at later times also provides increasingly greater reinforcement and greater motivation and retention. The reinforcement that takes place at a later time can take the form of additional comments from the nurse-teacher or opportunities for repetition of the successful experience.

PREDICTIVE PRINCIPLE: *Practice of learned activities in a variety of ways reinforces learned behaviors and promotes the ability to generalize and discriminate.*

Repetition of the same materials over and over again has little value for learning beyond habit fixation. Repetition, to be valuable, must have an improvement aspect. When repetition contains an improvement aspect, it becomes practice. Accompaniment of each repetition of the behavior by a feedback and correction cycle enables the learner to improve, if only slightly, each time he performs the behavior.

Repetition and overlearning are necessary for the purpose of achieving skill. Beyond achieving the required skill, repetition of learned behaviors in the same manner or in a similar situation is unnecessary and adds nothing to the learner's knowledge or skill.

Learning experiences spaced to allow the time lapses necessary for maturation are most effective for promoting retention. Rapid repetition of activities within a short period of time increases skill in narrow or single applications but contributes little to the learner's ability to generalize and discriminate.

Providing the learner with situations that require extraction of central principles and application of these principles to several problems or learning situations does three things: (1) it requires the learner to recognize and extract the central and uniting themes of situations (conceptualization); (2) it requires the application of principles to like situations (generalization); and (3) it requires the learner to perceive variables and make decisions and judgments about the selection of principles to apply to a given situation (evaluation and discrimination). An example of this type of reinforcement can be seen in the learner who had learned that microorganisms can move rapidly through moisture, which was an important consideration when sterile dressings were changed. Opportunities to work in other situations where sterile fields were important enabled her to extract selected central uniting concepts and principles of asepsis. The preparation of injections and emptying and changing urethral catheter drainage bags required that she select and apply the applicable aseptic commonalities discriminately.

Practice, either spaced or continuing, or applications to similar situations require periodic review, supervision, or evaluation by the learner and the teacher to ensure continued quality behaviors.

ESTABLISHING THE LEARNING ENVIRONMENT

The learning environment is not so much a matter of architecture as a matter of atmosphere. The building, patient units, classrooms, conference and office spaces, lighting, temperature, air circulation, paint color, piped-in music, and intercommunication systems affect the teaching-learning process to some degree.

Physical environment can facilitate teaching and learning through technologic aids, convenience, and comfort. However, the teacher with something to teach and the imagination, enthusiasm, and will to teach and the student who has the need, ability, and determination to learn will create an environment where teaching and learning can take place regardless of the surroundings.

Authority figures in the teaching-learning situation in health agencies set the tone and atmosphere for learning. However, learners are equally important contributors to the learning environment. The learner who brings negativism into the learning situation as a predominant characteristic can negate efforts of the nurse-teacher to establish an environment conducive to learning. Mutual contributions and consistent effort to create and maintain a positive learning environment are required of all participants. The nurse-teacher sets the pattern for learning interactions by implementing principles of teaching and learning that elicit positive responses from the patients, co-workers, and ancillary workers who are the learners.

PRINCIPLE: *A reciprocal relationship of trust and security facilitates teacher-learner communication and allows accurate assessment, learner participation in goal setting, and better utilization of resources.*

The optimal learning environment is basically one in which freedom is fostered by mutual trust. This allows the learner (1) the freedom to question without feeling foolish or stupid; (2) the freedom to participate in decisions; (3) the freedom of choice when there is a choice; (4) the freedom to learn as much as possible; and (5) the freedom to establish own goals and obtain help in reaching them. These are important freedoms in learning, and either the teacher or learner can alter the learning climate and decrease learning potential by tampering with the trust on which the learning freedoms exist.

Accurate assessment, learner participation in goal setting, and full utilization of resources are possible only if the teacher has self-trust. If the knowledge of self as a competent, adequate nurse depends upon knowing all answers and solutions to nursing problems, then the nurse-leader will not have the ability to participate freely in the teaching-learning process. Lack of self-trust can cause the nurse-teacher to guide learners only into content areas in which the teacher feels secure. This lack of self-trust places a rigid restriction on both content and method. (For a further discussion of self-trust, see Chapter 3.)

PRINCIPLE: *Recognition of the effect environment has on learning enables the nurse-teacher to mobilize environmental factors for the reinforcement of content.*

The physical environment and the climate in which learning takes place have a major effect on all phases of learning, and the inclusion of environmental considerations in teaching plans will help determine what is learned. Nurse-teachers often comment, "She knows better; why doesn't she do it?" The factors causing a discrepancy between what an individual "knows to do" and what he "does" are not specifically known. It is known that all behavior is meaningful, though not always understandable, and all behaviors are in response to some internal or external stimulus. The most usual approach to a solution of this problem is for the nurse-teacher to attack the overt behavior when some simple alteration in the forces that cause the behavior could enable real learning to take place.

Teacher behavior frequently exerts more influence on learning environment than does the material being taught. Following is an example of behavioral influence on the learning environment:

> A nurse-leader was orienting two new ancillary workers. After describing their duties, the leader assigned them to care for two patients and told them, "If you have any questions or are in doubt at all, just come and ask me." Later, when they did ask for information from the leader, the nurse answered the questions, but by her behavior she communicated impatience at being interrupted, and the ancillary workers felt stupid for asking questions. The verbal response was clear and simple; it was the behavior that communicated negatively. The ancillary workers sought no more help from the nurse-leader because her behavior created an environment that taught them not to ask when in doubt.

Contradictions between content and climate and lack of congruity between words and behavior cause confusion, and learners will respond to the clearest or least threatening message.

PRINCIPLE: *Making it explicit that accountability for learning rests with the learner enables the learner to meet his own learning needs and goals and enables the teacher to act as resource person, facilitator, validator, conferee, and consultant.*

PREDICTIVE PRINCIPLE: *Verbal or written contracts with client-learners for attainment of specific learner needs enable the nurse-teacher to enact the teaching role more explicitly and establish success criteria in collaboration with the learner.*

The nurse is in the peculiar position of being employed (usually) by an agency yet being the servant of the client. As in any profession, the professional loyalty of the nurse belongs to the client. Seldom do the nurse's allegiances to the client and to the employing agency conflict. For in health-related fields the objectives of all who deal in health are geared to attaining and maintaining or retaining the highest possible health level. Teaching needs of clients do sometimes cause some conflicts, since hospitalization of a patient may not be timed for the best possible prime teaching time, and teaching needs may span the involvement of several agencies. There are several ways around this problem, but none of them are entirely satisfactory and get at the problem created by the nurse's being agency based rather than client based. Some of these ways are discussed below.

1. *Involvement of the learner.* The nurse-teacher involves the learner to such a great extent that he assumes the responsibility for his own learning program. Continuity then rests with him. The client collaborates with the nurse, who makes the placement of responsibility explicit and helps him establish what he needs and wants to learn to solve his health problems. Together they attempt to establish alternative ways he might go about learning and establishing check points or criteria for measuring progress. The client can then call in other nurses,

other resource people or agencies, his public health nurse, or his physician for help in carrying out his learning program.

2. *Use of learning contracts.* A second alternative for solving this problem is through the use of learning contracts. Once the learning program is established, the nurse and client enter into a learning contract that incorporates both content and time so that mastery of specific content is completed within certain time constraints. Mastery of content is recognized by the attainment of certain specific criteria. Mastery means the ability to perform up to some established standard considered to be within the parameters of safety or desirability by both the nurse and the client.

3. *Continuity of care on a contractual basis.* Some acute agency-based nurses have a third alternative. They can, with agency support, incorporate so that they can follow patients into their homes on a fee-for-service basis to insure continuity of nursing care. This makes them available for helping the family and the patient and makes teaching continuity possible.

4. *Continuum of care on a donated basis.* Nurses often follow patients into their homes or other agencies on their own time. Having entered into a contract with a patient whose time constraints in a given agency did not permit closure of the learning episode, the nurse uses time off to conclude the contract. Care-oriented nurses find it satisfying, yet this activity overextends them. Nurses who make a practice of this should see their tax consultant to determine deductibility of donated time.

PREDICTIVE PRINCIPLE: *Structure, limits, and feedback provide an environment that promotes security and trust.*

Structure does not mean control or restricting the independence of the learner. Quite the contrary, structure is often the mechanism for providing for learning independence. Structure simply means to provide support, guidelines, and roadmaps for learning. Often all the learner wants or needs is someone to validate his learning or perceptions. Establishing a mechanism for validation is a form of structure. The balance between structure and nonstructure is delicate and difficult to maintain. However, it is essential to the learner's independence, creativity, and own need system to provide him with some sense of the parameters of environment (e.g., time constraints and the type of learning aids available) and the perameters of his learning needs (value of knowing certain things or behaviors).

Structure in the form of telling the learner what is going to happen, what is expected from the learner, what the acceptable limits are, the specific time limitations, and what the learner can expect from the nurse-teacher in teacher-student relationships and guidance provides a secure learning environment and decreases anxiety. Terms such as "positive environment," "freedom," "trust," and "security" need not be equated with lack of limits and structure. Lack of structure promotes insecurity, fear, and inhibition—not the desired security, trust, and freedom.

Structure in the form of specific learning objectives, limits, available learning experiences, expected relationships, and requirements for success provides a secure environment, which promotes learning. Comments such as, "I never really knew where I was with that nurse; I did not know what I was supposed to do or what was expected of me," indicate distrust, caused by a lack of the structure necessary for optimal learning.

LEARNING ACTIVITIES

All nurse-teachers utilize activities in teaching, whether by accident or intention. Activities are all those things that will make learning take place. Activities can involve people, agencies, books, charts, or any source of content; they can be projects, audiovisual aids, or any teaching tool. Thus, learning activities enable acquisition of knowledge and recall; they reinforce, promote, transfer, and foster generalizations and discrimination. The planning of learning activities for the maximum benefit of the learner will insure efficient accomplishment of behavioral objectives.

PREDICTIVE PRINCIPLE: *The more frames of reference (learning theories) the nurse-teacher is able to use, the more teaching strategies will be in his teaching repertoire.*

There are many theories of learning. This book presents only two—behaviorism and cognitivism. These two frames of reference are at opposite ends of the learning compendium. Behaviorism is sometimes called stimulus-response associationism. Whereas classic conditioning deals with inevitable, or reflex, responses, operant conditioning deals with voluntary behavior. Other names for operant conditioning based on behaviorist learning theory are instrumental conditioning and behavior modification. When the desired response occurs, whether accidental or guided, a reward meaningful to the learner is provided so that the probability of the desired response reoccurring is increased. The basic thesis of operant conditioning is that the frequency with which any act occurs may be altered by the consequence of the act.

Gestalt field theory or cognitive field theory has as its salient feature that man in his environment is a unit participating in what is called a simultaneous mutual interaction. This theory of learning conceives of perception as all the different ways one becomes familiar with his environment and not mere consciousness of his environment. Things and people are perceived differently by different individuals because their perception depends on the sum total of their life experiences and how they perceive other things in their life space concomitantly. (Whereas stimulus-response associationism emphasizes single units— one organism [human being], one stimulus, and one response—and an effective reinforcer, cognitive field theory deals with the concept of person [meaning the individual] within his whole field.) Cognitive field theory proposes that hypotheses which help to determine causal interrelationships and organize facts to provide direction and predictability are the heart of a science. Reality for the cognitivist is what that individual perceives and experiences it to be for himself. Nothing exists in and of itself to people; things exist in relationship to a person's total experience. The cognitivist theory has the following characteristics:

1. Insight
2. Putting things together to make a pattern

3. Seeing things in relationship to each other (For example, sickness can only be viewed in relation to health; passive can only be viewed in relation to active; and happiness can only be viewed in relation to sadness.)
4. Always developing

Other theoretical frames of reference for learning can be derived from learning-theory source books. Several are given in the bibliography. Since the nurse-leader has a teaching role, one of the tasks essential to role development is an exploration of learning theories. The nurse-leader can from this base develop a useful eclectic approach to teaching-learning situations.

PREDICTIVE PRINCIPLE: *Learning episodes that contain input, operations, and feedback increase retention and utility of learning.*

Learning is a change in behavior that is acquired as a result of practice and that can be repeated when the need is aroused.

Learning has three identifiable aspects that exist regardless of the learning theory adopted:

1. An input aspect
2. An operation aspect
3. A feedback aspect

These aspects are variously called sequences or phases, but since both sequence and phase imply a serial order in time, "aspects" is used here, for aspects can occur simultaneously. Graphically, learning is like a pyramid with three sides, one each for input, operation, and feedback.

1. *Input* is the acquisition of information and the organization of the information into action hypotheses (predictive principles). These activities may be assessments, content information, instructions, recognition that a response is appropriate, or any of the *cognitive* activities associated with acquiring input.
2. *Operation* is the *activity phase;* it is directly observable behavior, responses to the input and interactions. It is practice (prescriptive theory). In memorization it is repetition (either oral or written). In discovery learning it is testing out ideas, either by putting them into action or interacting with another person. The operation aspect is *response.*
3. *Feedback* is the result of the operational test or the result of evaluation. The feedback becomes input that confirms, alters, changes, or refutes the cognitive phase or input.

The three aspects of a learning episode frequently occur with such speed that clear delineation between aspects is not always possible. For instance, the operational place is in effect a test or trial or acting out of the input. The very act of doing generates immediate "fingertip" feedback that becomes input for corrections. The most useful element about familiarity with the three phases is that the presence of all three phases in any learning episode increases the likelihood of the learner actually having a change of behavior.

PREDICTIVE PRINCIPLE: *The more teaching strategies and operations available to and useable by the nurse-teacher, the better able the nurse-teacher will be to select a strategy based on learner and situational needs.*

Choosing a teaching strategy is dependent upon several variables. Most of these variables are simple logical ways of looking at the factors governing the means by which the learner and the teacher can find a common learning medium. If the learner is a patient in the hospital or home, consideration must be given to his mobility, his energy level, the availability of resources (books, pamphlets, audiovisual materials), the content to be taught, the amount of anxiety surrounding the teaching subject, and the number of other stimuli being received by the patient and his family. Families and other people significant to the client have a part in choosing the learning strategies if they are going to participate in the learning episode.

Most teaching strategies are passive in nature. The learner reads, watches, and listens. These teaching strategies provide the major modality for cognitive input. They will probably continue to remain a central learning modality because early in a human's life, reading, listening, and watching play prominent roles in gathering information. People seldom simply experiment and rediscover information each time it is needed—that method is too inefficient. Many advances in modern technology assist learning—television, super 8 millimeter film, tape cassettes, telephone dialing information systems, film strips, slides, programmed books, transparencies, and the whole gamut of audiovisual materials, which bring information to learners in a wide variety of formats. These informational packages can be put together in learning modules tailor-made for learner and situational idiosyncrasies. The bibliography for this chapter contains references to resources helpful to the nurse who wishes to make multimedia learning modules for clients or other health care givers.

The nurse-leader who teaches the same or similar content repeatedly to clients may wish to make, or work with the agency to purchase, learning modules using several media as the input mode for selected clients. Other patients, depending upon their cognitive style, may wish to participate in the development of an individualized program of study, complete a programmed text designed to meet their needs, or may wish simply to read or listen to the nurse-teacher talk with them about the content.

The operation sequence of learning demands that the learner *do* something with the information. This activity may involve solving a simulated problem, practicing a procedure, recalling, building, creating, making, using, or any other active operationalization of the input (information). The act of *doing* provides a basis for the feedback sequence. Feedback arises not only from the formal evaluative material available on tests but also from the act itself. As learners practice or get involved in some utilization of information, the information begins to correct itself, make further sense, fit into patterns, and make generalization insights possible.

Each phase of the learning process—input, operation, and feedback—needs to be devised in collaboration with the learner and chosen for its ability to meet his specific needs and the needs of the situation in which he finds himself during learning.

Simulation teaching techniques offer the nurse-leader an opportunity to develop teaching skills with exciting dimensions. Usually health teaching involves information giving, demonstration, and return demonstration. Creative teaching strategies provide the client-learner, the co-worker-learner, and the nurse-leader the opportunity to experience behaviors that are the objectives of the learning episode. For instance, the nursing care giver who is teaching the child-diabetic to give insulin often uses a syringe, a bottle of water, and a lemon or orange, or a sponge specially designed for this purpose. This technique is a form of simulation. Role playing a patient interview with a colleague provides the nurse with alternative approaches and interviewing behaviors that are difficult to learn in the real situation. Children learning balanced dietary habits are sometimes given models of food to put on a plate for a balanced meal. These forms of simulation provide practice when the "real thing" cannot be studied directly because it is too expensive, not available, or is too dangerous.

Children and adults enjoy playing games, and games lend themselves well to learning. Games are contests requiring skill or luck. Skill or good memory retention can provide the nurse with the structure for a game. Bingo provides a model for a game to aid memorization, as is needed for classification of foodstuffs or vitamin content. Guessing games such as "my ship comes in sailing" and "20 questions" are models for information games. Problem games where players are given a diabetic insulin and food balance problem make good learning exercises. The reader is referred to the bibliography for resource materials concerning game theory and utilization.

PREDICTIVE PRINCIPLE: *Utilization of problem-solving processes promotes continuity and ease of learning.*

A knowledge of the problem-solving process is a learner skill that promotes a systematic use of appropriate resources. Problem solving takes place in many ways; however, the more systematic the problem-solving, the more reliable the result. The neophyte in systematic problem solving will find a logical format or model contributes to his skill. The following is a suggested guideline for problem solving in tasks or stages.

Stage I, problem identification or establishment of objectives, is the initial task and the keystone of problem solving. Stage II is the gathering of appropriate data or the selection of appropriate principles. This stage requires (1) a survey of all the learner or problem-solver knows about the problem, (2) a collection of the antecedent knowledge patterned into concepts, and (3) formulation of the concepts into predictive principles. These predictive principles enable the learner to list possible alternatives of action (stage III). Stage IV, a listing of the risks inherent in each alternative, helps the learner to make a logical choice of alternatives, choosing the one that has the greatest chance of solving the problem with the least chance of damaging the patient or the situation. An additional stage (stage V), in which all possible applications of the theories, facts, concepts, and principles used in the problem are listed, will be useful as an aid to further generalizations. The additional stage will also help the learner or problem-solver to reinforce learning. Utilizing problem-solving processes in a tangible form can make content logical and sensible to the learner. Use of such methodology will provide an overview of all elements of the content.

Since much of nursing and health maintenance is applied science, health

Problem-solving sample*

STATEMENT OF PROBLEM OBJECTIVE	NECESSARY FACTS OR CONCEPTS	PRINCIPLES[†]
PROBLEM How to get the LVN to use appropriate mouth care with two critically ill patients who were N.P.O. and mouth breathers.	1. Mouth is the portal of entry for food. 2. Digestion is started in the mouth, where food is thoroughly chewed and mixed with saliva, which contains the digestive enzyme ptyalin.	A. A well cared for mouth during critical illness increases the patient's ability to return to normal eating habits upon recovery (1). B. A sensitive or infected mouth produces discomfort (2). (Food is often swallowed before it is thoroughly chewed and mixed with saliva or food may not be eaten at all.)
OBJECTIVE The licensed vocational nurse (LVN) is (1) able to select the correct type of mouth care for each patient and (2) able to give adequately the correct type of mouth care to meet the individual needs of each patient.	3. If the jaws are not used for mastication and if there is no acid or alkaline intake, there is little or no stimulation of parotid secretion. 4. Salivary flow is decreased in severe illness. 5. Salivary flow has a constant cleansing action. 6. Anaerobic organisms do not ordinarily grow in the mouth. 7. The accumulation of dried secretions in the mouth provides an environment conducive to the growth of anaerobic organisms. 8. When the mouth is dry, local treatment with fluids and emollients gives temporary relief. 9. Application of lemon juice and glycerine to the tongue and gums is a classic treatment for dry mouth. 10. State of hydration of the patient is not dependent upon the moisture of the mucous membranes of the mouth.	C. N.P.O. causes the parotid glands to become inactive (3). D. Meticulous mouth care prevents the massive invasion of microorganisms from the mouth through the parotid duct to the inactive gland(s) (3, 11). E. Decreased salivary flow creates the need for frequent and special mouth care (4). F. Local treatment of dry mouth with fluid and emollients promotes temporary relief (5). G. The use of lemon juice for special mouth care causes an increased secretion of saliva (5, 7, 8, 9). H. The use of hydrogen peroxide, an oxidizing agent, for mouth care inhibits the growth of anaerobic organisms in the mouth (7). I. The use of hydrogen peroxide for mouth care results in a bubbling action that facilitates the removal of undesirable excretions in the mouth (8). J. The use of concentrated glycerine alone (which is hydroscopic) for special mouth care predisposes to dehydration and irritation of mouth tissues (9, 12, 13). K. Small amounts of glycerine promote softening and protect mucous membranes (9, 12, 13).

*This problem is the work of Honor B. Dufour and is used with her permission.
[†]Numbers after principles refer to number of facts or concepts used to compose it.
[‡]Letters after statements refer to principles used to devise action.

PRESCRIPTIONS[‡]	POSSIBLE RISKS INVOLVED	GENERALIZATIONS
Frequent examination of the mouth to ascertain its condition. Observe for dryness, collection of undesirable excretions, redness, and odor. If patient is responsive, question him concerning subjective condition of his mouth—discomfort, pain, difficulty swallowing, foul taste (A, B, C).	Examination may be incomplete because of poor visibility. A tongue blade may be necessary to hold tongue down during examination, but care must be taken *not* to damage delicate tissues. Patient may not give dependable answers to questions.	This procedure for special mouth care would be applicable to any patient in whom the salivary flow is decreased. Some common examples would be: Patient who is comatose Patient suffering from severe dehydration Patient unable to swallow Patient receiving oxygen therapy
Use tongue blade and light when necessary to improve visualization of oral cavity (A, B, C).	Aspirating agent used for oral care.	Patient with collection of foul debris in the mouth Patient who is N.P.O. Patient receiving chemical therapy that has drying effect on the mouth *Discrimination:* This procedure would *not* be applicable in any situation where blood clots were necessary for healing (oral surgery).
Give mouth care with lemon juice and glycerine if there is danger of the patient swallowing the substances (E, F, G, J, K). Careful positioning of patient with head to one side to prevent aspiration; such machine should be available if patient is not responsive or cooperative (O).	Glycerine must not be too concentrated, since it can be dehydrating and irritating. The nurse must obtain help to position the patient if he cannot do it alone. If suctioning is required, care must be taken *not* to damage delicate tissues.	

Continued.

Problem-solving sample—cont'd

STATEMENT OF PROBLEM OBJECTIVE	NECESSARY FACTS OR CONCEPTS	PRINCIPLES
LVN able to select and give correct mouth care—cont'd	11. Antiseptic rinses stimulate saliva flow and decrease microorganism population. 12. Gylcerine (concentrated) is hydroscopic and is a drying agent. 13. Small amounts of glycerine can protect and soften. 14. Excretions such as dried blood, mucus, and sputum in the mouth may be removed by the use of hydrogen peroxide, which is an oxidizing agent. 15. Saliva putrefies rapidly, giving rise to objectionable odors. 16. Water is not effective in removing odors. 17. Substances such as petroleum jelly and cocoa butter applied to the lips and tongue have a protective action. 18. Mechanical action and friction remove dried and putrefied materials and stimulate salivation. 19. Cleaning patient's mouth while he is positioned on back makes it easy for patient to aspirate.	L. Use of an antiseptic mouth wash results in lessening of halitosis (11, 13, 14, 15). M. Petroleum jelly applied to the lips and tongue after special mouth care results in a slower drying of these tissues (17). N. Careful use of mechanics and scrubbing promotes removal of dried blood, mucus, and sputum (18). O. Positioning of patient on side during mouth care promotes drainage of secretions outward and prevents aspiration (19).

teachers frequently draw facts, concepts, and principles from the basic sciences of anatomy, physiology, chemistry, bacteriology, physics, and the social sciences. Often the student has difficulty in seeing the relationship between these antecedents and his goal. The nurse-teacher who begins the teaching process with the basic science concepts may lose the learner because he does not see the antecedent-goal relationship. Conversely, teachers who initiate the process with the application or "nursing action" phase may lose the learner because he does not understand the antecedent information that supplies the "why."

Objectives can be realized when the teacher and learner participate together in the problem-solving process using a simple graphic model so that individual parts of knowledge can be patterned into a meaningful whole. The above is an example of a problem-solving tool in which the hygiene activity of mouth care has been chosen as the subject. The topic chosen is simply to enable emphasis to be placed upon the process and not the content. The above example can be used as a model and can be successfully employed for any content regardless of complexity. The goal may be stated as a behavioral objective or as a problem,

PRESCRIPTIONS	POSSIBLE RISKS INVOLVED	GENERALIZATIONS
	Hydrogen peroxide can injure the gums if used improperly, may cause gingival hypertrophy if used over a long period of time.	
	Hydrogen peroxide not diluted to a strength of about 1% can injure tissues.	
If the mouth is foul with dried blood, mucus, and sputum, use hydrogen peroxide to remove crusts, followed with antiseptic mouth wash and then apply petroleum jelly to lips and the tongue (unless the patient complains of the taste) (E, H, I, L, M).	Oils, such as mineral oil, are contraindicated because of the danger of aspiration and the development of lipoid pneumonia or lung abscess.	
	All special mouth care performed with inappropriate tools can injure tissues or be ineffective in accomplishing goals. Applicators are rarely effective.	
Special mouth care is best carried out with a toothbrush; however, in some instances a protected forceps and soft gauze sponges may be substituted (N).	If protected forceps are used, care must be taken not to injure the buccal tissues or disturb oral injury, surgery, or dental work.	

depending upon which is appropriate to the situation. Both a behavioral objective and a stated problem are given below for clarity and to demonstrate the flexiblity of the tool.

Problem-solving sample

Either a problem or a behavioral objective requires the learner to have knowledge of facts, theories, concepts, principles, and risks involved so that he may generalize, discriminate, and perform to accomplish the objective or solve the problem.

The process enables the nurse-teacher to identify all the knowledge relevant to the development of a module or small unit of teaching. Once the necessary components of the sample model are identified, the nurse-teacher can share the overall pattern with the learner, and through learner participation can select knowledge that (1) does not need to be covered, (2) needs to be reviewed, and (3) needs to be learned. In this way the teacher can start where the learner is and utilize what the learner brings into the learning situation. Once the content is selected, the methods, teaching tools, and other resources to be used can be chosen or devised. Use of the tool itself as a single method rather than as an overall guide stereotypes teaching and develops rigidity, which can decrease the creative enthusiasm in teaching and learning.

PRINCIPLE: *Content that flows from the familiar to the unfamiliar provides a point of reference and promotes efficient grasping of material.*

The learner is the nurse-teacher's greatest resource. The teacher who assesses what the learner knows, not only about the subject in question but about other areas of interest to him, can relate this familiar knowledge to the unknown.

For example, a maintenance worker in a factory that used steam boilers suffered a heart attack. Arteriosclerotic heart disease was diagnosed. The community health nurse used the patient's knowledge of the precipitation of mineral content of water in boilers and pipes and the resultant dangers of clogging and pressure in the boiler system to teach the patient about arteriosclerosis, blood pressure, and myocardial infarcts.

It is not always possible to teach material from the "simple" to the "complex" because "simple" and "complex" are relative terms to the learner and actually depend upon what related knowledge and experience the learner brings to the learning situation.

EVALUATION

Evaluation is the bugaboo of all those engaged in the teaching-learning process. Evaluation is the process through which the teacher and the learner determine progress toward the learning objective.

Evaluation for the purpose of establishing a "grade" may only tell the learner his achievement as rated on some established scale and usually compares him to other learners attempting to master the same content. Evaluation should be for the purpose of providing the learner with a guide that will enable him to determine his progress toward accomplishing a desired goal. It should help him ascertain his goal achievement. This latter purpose is best suited to health teaching and problem solving, since the evaluation goal is to assess behavioral changes in relationship to the goal or defined problem.

Evaluation for better learning enables the nurse-teacher and the learner to determine (1) that a desired behavior has or has not been learned and (2) how well a desired behavior has been learned.

Quantitative evaluation is of little use to the nurse-leader. Quantitative evaluations are characterized by words like *always, frequently, sometimes, rarely,* and *never. Qualitative* evaluations are characterized by descriptions of behaviors that indicate the stage the learner has reached in the theory-building or problem-solving process and how skilled he has become in that stage. Qualitative evaluations tell the character and nature of success or failure.

An example of the differences in quantitative and qualitative evaluations can be drawn from the situation in which the nurse-leader was teaching an elderly man to administer injections to his wife who had pernicious anemia. The man had extreme difficulty in manipulating the syringe and vial without contamination. The nurse's evaluative note, which states, "very rarely draws up solution correctly" and "frequently contaminates the syringe" does not convey to either the teacher or the learner what has or has not been accomplished. A qualitative evaluative statement would read, "has identified the components of aseptic technique but has difficulty with the coordination necessary to master the handling of the vial and syringe without contamination. He is aware of breaks in techniques and is developing manipulative skills slowly." This statement conveys specifically and clearly the stage of learning achieved in behavioral terms.

PRINCIPLE: *Objectives expressed as learner behaviors enable the teacher and learner to know the limits of expected outcomes and to evaluate in meaningful, specific terms.*

The time required to write detailed behavioral objectives is compensated for by the efficiency with which one can plan the content necessary to accomplish the objective and the ease with which behavioral objectives can be evaluated. Behavioral objectives definitely describe the precise activities necessary to demonstrate that the desired learnings have occurred. For example, the practical nurse who was learning aseptic technique would not know what was expected of her if she were trying to achieve the objective: "to become increasingly knowledgeable about aseptic technique." "Knowledgeable" does not indicate what behaviors result from the knowledge. Contrastingly, "to be able to recognize when aseptic technique is required" and "to perform tasks requiring aseptic technique in any situation" are two objectives that tell the learner and teacher exactly what behaviors must be achieved to accomplish the objective. It spells out criteria for both teacher and learner to use in judging accomplishment.

The above principle indicates that evaluation in meaningful and specific terms is an activity of both teacher and learner. Evaluation carried out by either, exclusive of the other, reduces the effectiveness of the evaluation by making it impossible for one half of the teaching-learning team to use the evaluation in activities designed for further goal accomplishment. For successful evaluation both teacher and learner profit by having the data necessary to assess the present situation and to structure additional experiences for achievement of the desired behavioral changes.

APPLICATION OF PRINCIPLES OF TEACHING AND LEARNING

Mr. Scarborough, a 34-year-old alert man, has acute thrombophlebitis of the right leg. He is on complete bed rest with his legs wrapped with Ace bandages to midthigh (rewrap q4h), heat cradle to lower extremities, and anticoagulant therapy. One of the aides reported to the nurse-leader that she had seen Mr. Scarborough twisting a towel tightly around his right thigh. When the aide asked him why, Mr. Scarborough stated, "It eases the pain."

PROBLEM	PRINCIPLES	COURSE OF ACTION
How to teach Mr. Scarborough healthful ways of alleviating the pain of thrombophlebitis	The learner's developmental stage, personal characteristics, and prior experiences influence learning potential and dictate content.	Assess prior experiences, previous knowledge, and personal characteristics. *Continued.*

PROBLEM	PRINCIPLES	COURSE OF ACTION
To teach ways of alleviating pain—cont'd	The learner's prevalent life needs determines what he will learn.	Use learner need to decrease pain as starting point.
	A reciprocal relationship of trust and security facilitates teacher-learner communication and allows accurate asessment, learner participation in goal setting, and better utilization of resources.	Establish open and trustful communication using activities conducive to establishing trust and open communication.
	Participation of the learner in setting learning goals increases the number of learning activities meaningful and useful to the learner.	Collaborate (his need and nurse's specialized knowledge and skill) in establishing learning goals in behavioral terms; that is, identify a variety of methods for reducing the pain without jeopardizing his health; choose the appropriate method for each situation; perform the activities necessary to the implementation of the chosen alternative.
	An obvious relationship between learning activities and stated goals increases the motivational value of the activity.	Develop a brief overview of necessary content in collaboration with patient.
	Rewards consistent with the valve system of the learner such as recognition, praise, peer status, or valued gains are motivating and reinforcing influences and thus facilitate learning rate, amount of retention, and degree of behavior change.	Determine appropriate rewards and use as reinforcers.
	Utilization of problem-solving processes promotes continuity and ease of learning.	Use flexible approach building toward a useful body of predictive principles based on valid antecedents.
	Content that flows from the familiar to the unfamiliar provides a point of reference and promotes efficient grasping of material.	Use meaningful similes (based on prior experiences), such as, a clogged drain causes drainage backup and overflow and collection of solids at point of obstruction, causing further clogging.
	Objectives expressed as learner behaviors enable the teacher and learner to know the limits of expected outcomes and to evaluate in meaningful, specific terms.	Evaluate patient's ability to behave in the manner specified above and thereby gain relief from the pain. If possible, reinforce behavior; if not possible, determine with patient what would be necessary steps for achievement of success.

BIBLIOGRAPHY

Babcock, S. S., and Schild, E. O.: Simulation games in learning, Beverly Hills, Calif., 1968, Sage Publications, Inc.

Barton, R. E.: A primer on simulation and gaming, Englewood Cliffs, N. J., 1970, Prentice-Hall, Inc.

Begge, M.: Learning theories for teachers, ed. 2, New York, 1971, Harper & Row, Publishers.

Biehler, R. F.: Psychology applied to teaching, New York, 1971, Houghton Mifflin Co.

Biehler, R. F.: Psychology applied to teaching: selected readings, New York, 1971, Houghton Mifflin Co.

Bower, F. L.: The process of planning nursing care, a theoretical model, St. Louis, 1972, The C. V. Mosby Co.

Carlson, E.: Learning through games, Washington, D. C., 1968, Public Affairs Press.

De Tornyay, R.: Strategies for teaching nursing, New York, 1971, John Wiley & Sons, Inc.

Erikson, E. H.: Childhood and society, ed. 2, New York, 1963, W. W. Norton & Co., Inc.

Glasser, W.: Schools without failure, New York, 1969, Harper & Row, Publishers.

Havelock, R. G.: A guide to innovation in education, Ann Arbor, Mich., 1970, Institute for Social Research, The University of Michigan.

Interaction Associates: Strategy notebook, San Francisco, 1971, Interaction Associates, Inc.

Lefrancois, G. R.: Psychology for teaching, a bear always faces the front, Belmont, Calif., 1972, Wadsworth Publishing Co., Inc.

McDonald, F. J.: Educational psychology, Melmont, Calif., 1966, Wadsworth Publishing Co., Inc.

Mosston, M.: Teaching: from command to discovery, Belmont, Calif., 1972, Wadsworth Publishing Co., Inc.

Rogers, C.: Freedom to learn, Columbus, Ohio, 1969, Charles E. Merrill Publishing Co.

Schrank, J.: Teaching human beings: 101 subversive activities for the classroom, Boston, 1972, Beacon Press.

Shaffer, S. M., Indorato, K. L., and Deneselya, J. A.: Teaching in schools of nursing, St. Louis, 1972, The C. V. Mosby Co.

Wilson, S. F., and Tosti, D. T.: Learning is getting easier, 1972, Individual Learning Systems, Inc.

CHAPTER THREE

Predictive principles of effective communication: interpersonal and groups

PERCEPTION OF SELF AND OTHERS

The value systems of the leader and the group influence the establishment of goals and the setting of priorities and govern the amount of effort given to goal attainment.

Continuity of competent leadership facilitates the efficiency of communication process.

Characteristics of client and nurse-leader determine the type of communications that will evolve.

REINFORCEMENT AND FEEDBACK

Integrative positive reinforcement increases individual identification with group goals and the participation level of the individual.

Perceiving negative feedback enables group members to become aware of others' responses to them and their effects on the group and to evaluate goal attainment and to modify behavior accordingly.

The dependent, interdependent, and/or independent natures of relationships affect the structure of the communication process.

The interdependent collaborating group facilitates group goal accomplishment.

Continuing reference and clarification of goals enhance the ability to attain those goals.

COMMUNICATION STRATEGIES

The type of communications at work in a group predicts member perception and resultant action.

Congruent behavioral and verbal messages promote clear communication.

Threat and resulting anxiety, unless resolved, can inhibit individual and group functioning.

Questions and discussion geared to second and third level theories promote cognition that is more useful in nursing activities than questions and discussion geared to first and second level theories.

Use of simulation processes facilitates decision making and provides efficient means for learning problem-solving methods in a nonthreatening and safe environment.

GOAL SETTING, ACHIEVEMENT, AND EVALUATION

Preassessment of individual and group knowledges, skills, and expectations establishes baseline data for measurement of progress or change.

Mutual understanding and agreement on goals appropriate to the client or agency ensure support for goal achievement.

Circumstance and member capability determine the type of direction to be communicated.

Opportunity to express expectations of the individual or group, when translated into meaningful terms to members, relates directly to individual identification and invites commitment of members to goal achievement.

Realistic and valid goals promote achievement.

The extent of involvement of each group member determines the proficiency of the group.

Group involvement in goal setting necessitates the endorsement of the agency and commitment of membership to participate in the outcome.

EFFECTIVE CONFERENCES

Adequate preparation by the leader for all conferences expedites fulfillment of expectations for the conference.

Relieving care givers of responsibility while conference is in session allows members to proceed without interruption.

Prior announcement of time, place, purpose, and duration of conferences to all concerned promotes assembly of a group well prepared and ready to focus attention on the purposes of the conference.

DIRECTION-GIVING CONFERENCES

Obtaining the most recent data available prior to conference assures the leader that imparted information is pertinent, inclusive, and accurate.

Information to care givers and/or clients that is paced, systematic, and inclusive allows participants time to assimilate the content and provides them with information necessary to function.

PATIENT-CENTERED CONFERENCES

Interaction of conference members on an equal basis encourages active participation and leads to usable solutions to the problem.

Identification of the nursing problem to be considered expedites the formulation of nursing intervention.

Analyzing nursing care given in the light of established goals enables members to validate their behavior and to devise ways to improve nursing care.

Formation of written nursing care plans from patient-centered conferences provides a central, continuous source of information.

CONTENT CONFERENCES

Member participation in problem-solving processes during content conference results in desired knowledge being patterned into a meaningful whole.

Conferences held between nurse and client and/or significant others contribute to reciprocal development of care plans and lead to optimal health service for the client and satisfaction for the nurse.

Periodic care review conferences held with colleagues provide a mechanism for the nurse to validate care plans and maintain quality control.

REPORTING CONFERENCES

Directions given to conferees before report reveal expectations the leader has for the members.

GENERAL PROBLEMS CONFERENCES

Sharing of feelings through conferences unifies and integrates the membership and allows work to progress.

Understanding and management of group behavior require ability to predict the processes through which feelings and meanings are transmitted among group members.

Involvement in group process results in specific gains or losses for the individual member.

Nurses function in high stimulus environments, of which communications is a major source of excitants. Leadership, as defined in the theoretical framework, is a set of actions that influence members of a group to move toward common goal setting and attainment. There is simply no way communication skills can be separated from leadership abilities because the most usual mode of exercising leadership is through the interactive process, which uses communicating as a primary vehicle.

Communications is the sending, receiving, and validating of a message. According to rueschian theory, communications is the ability of one mind to affect another and includes all methods for transmitting and receiving messages— pictures, paintings, sculpture, music, dance, signs and signals, written and vocal, and extrasensory transmissions. However, for the process to be communication, one mind must indeed affect another and that impact must be sent, received, and validated. Therefore communications is circular; that is, it has a built-in feedback system. This chapter will deal with two basic types of communication, interpersonal and group. Basically the same factors influence communications in these two contexts with only minor differences.

Interpersonal communications follows the definition given above. A statement is an expressive action on the part of a sender. The statement can be an article, a series of sign-language signals, posture, body language, verbal statement, directions, or information. It can be a purposive expression of thoughts and feelings. But as long as the verbal or nonverbal language is one way, it is simply a statement and does not qualify as communications. When that purposive expression of personal thought or feelings has been perceived and interpreted by another individual, it is a message. When that message is acknowledged as received in any way whatsoever, it becomes interpersonal communication. To be perfected, the communication must be clarified or corrected. This is feedback, which allows the communication to change, modify, and clarify to bring the intent of the message sent into focus as the interpretation of the message received.

For feedback to be useful it must be properly timed, appropriate to the situation, and delivered in a clear, understandable way. Both negative and positive feedback play an important part in growth and stabilization of communications.

Group communications can refer to an individual and a group of people communicating with each other, or to a group of people communicating with another group. Usually in group communications, feedback and correction are slow, and change is more ponderous. Generally speaking, the more bureaucratic the system and the larger the group, the more slowly perception, response, and correction occur.

The purpose of group communications, like individual communications, is to enable collaboration in finding solutions to problems and meeting needs. This differs markedly from making statements and giving directions or providing information. These are one-way messages not geared to collaboration.

Communications break down for several reasons:

1. *Overloading the system.* Human communications share a characteristic with animal and machine communications; that is, overloading causes them to break down. A computer will click out on overload; an animal will show signs of purposeless or erratic behavior, motor-neuron synaptic failure, or other signs of "nervous breakdown." A human being will replace

normal modes of communication with private modes or will restrict communication to the intrapersonal system (talk to himself) or some other protective device. Reduction in the communication load and reduction of other stimuli are necessary for intervention and reestablishment of successful communicating patterns.

2. *Malfunction of the communication apparatus.* This can be from disease or from poor or insufficient mastery of the use of communication apparatuses (eyes, ears, and vocal ability).

3. *Incorrect information.* This is erroneous perception or interpretation of data, or faulty data. Anytime the input is faulty, the response will probably be defective.

4. *Misuse of or using too few communication strategies and tactics.* Strategies and tactics provide for the sending of messages and the obtaining and utilization of feedback.

Since practice in nursing is basically group and interpersonally oriented, people do not tend to work in a vacuum or alone. All types of nursing require collaboration with other health care givers or clients. Therefore much of this chapter will deal with group work. Leadership communications with groups are designed primarily to facilitate groups in the setting of goals and the activities necessary to the attainment of those goals.

Group work extends throughout all health services. Nurses are called upon routinely to work with groups of personnel who have a diversity of experience and preparation. The nurse should be able to operate in any structural care pattern (for example, case, functional, team, or primary) or within varied organizational systems established for provision of care.

In this context, group refers to a number of people, small or large, who work for a common purpose: that of providing quality of nursing care to a specific client or numbers of patients in any setting. Process refers to the goal-oriented operations of the group and to the forces at work within the operational procedure. For almost a quarter of a century the dynamics of group behavior has been studied intensely by psychologists, sociologists, and educators. The study of group process on a scientific basis is a relatively new field; hence there are no absolutes, but there are sufficient data to give indications of the processes most useful to leaders working with a number of people. Efforts to classify groups and to identify internal processes reveal that the general laws concerning group life, regardless of their nature, are applicable to all groups, large or small.

Nurses draw from the studies of various groups and from the body of knowledge acquired concerning group dynamics to formulate predictive principles useful in nursing practice. The following section is addressed to leaders who are utilizing communications in all phases of nursing. No attempt has been made to deal specifically with therapeutic communications; however, the predictive principles discussed have relevance to all phases of nursing.

PERCEPTION OF SELF AND OTHERS

Perceptions, like beauty, are in the eye of the beholder. The nurse's total self-system effects his perceptions. Value systems, ideals, life goals, experiences, presets, expectations of self and others, context—all affect perception. What a person sees and hears and how he interprets this information are regulated by the self-system. Perception is more than seeing and hearing; it also includes interpreting this data. Interpretations are functions of values, social conditioning, and life experiences and expectations. The leader's perception of himself affects his view of others. If the leader sees others with a positive preset, then that will affect other's responses to him and reaffirm his predeterminations. In other words, individuals who believe they will receive affirmative responses from people condition themselves to elicit positive responses because their approach to others is with this type of expectation. The converse is also true. People who expect negative reactions usually communicate behaviorally such expectations and elicit similar negative responses from the communicant.

Perceptions of others also affect communications. Leader perceptions of an individual or group are usually only parts of the true picture. The same is true of the group's or individual's perception of the leader. The invalidity or lack of authenticity in perception greatly influences interpretation of behavior and communication. Sharing insight about perceptions and self within the group will aid the efficiency of communication.

PRINCIPLE: *The leader's self-perception directly relates to the development of positive perceptions of each group member.*

Since much of the leadership role is individual and personal, the role demands employment of self as an instrument and involvement as a person. It is essential that the leader have both the ability to share himself as well as the capacity for self-discipline. Perceptual psychologists have indicated the deeply deprived self cannot afford to give itself away. The self must possess a satisfactory degree of adequacy before it can venture commitment to and provide encounter with individuals or groups. Leadership is dependent upon entering into an interaction relationship with others, and effective leaders possess sufficient self-esteem to make sharing and supporting relationships possible. The nurse-leader needs to feel personally adequate to deal effectively with others.

The effective leader believes himself fundamentally adequate, which enables him to give adequate attention to client and care giver's needs. Those who feel inadequate and deprived cannot afford the time and effort required to lead and assist others. In the University of Florida studies of the helping professions a number of perceptual psychologists studied the nature of self-fulfillment and personal adequacy in professional leaders and directors. It was found that effective leaders felt themselves being (1) identified with rather than apart from others, (2) basically adequate rather than inadequate, (3) trustworthy rather than untrustworthy, (4) wanted rather than unwanted or ignored, and (5) worthy rather than overlooked or discounted.

The nurse-leader who has a positive self-perception is able to provide necessary positive support and reinforcement to clients and members of the health team. The nurse-leader with positive perceptions of self communicates positive perceptions of themselves to others, thereby increasing the self-esteem of individuals and group members. With the self-concept strengthened, participants can in turn often develop into support agents for other relationships, as, for example, with clients.

PREDICTIVE PRINCIPLE: *The value systems of the leader and the group influence the establishment of goals and the setting of priorities and govern the amount of effort given to goal attainment.*

Value systems are those ethics, ideas, objects, behaviors, or philosophies important to an individual. Value systems are outgrowths of life experiences, life goals, ambitions, and ethnic background. Values dictate the moral, ethical, material, and religious "set" of individuals. The leader and every member bring to their group a value system. The sum total of this pooling of values is an amorphous group personality. Because of the makeup of a group and of its climate, leadership, and task, the group's value system becomes evident in what is important to it, that is, in what receives its attention and efforts. Changes perceived by the leader and the group as having great worth will receive high priorities and much effort, while changes or goals viewed by the group as unimportant or of little value will receive slight effort and be of low priority. Priority setting is a direct function of individual and group values.

If goals are established that the group does not value, usually the personnel will not work toward them. However, other extraneous factors may enter in. If rewards for goal achievement become important enough, receiving the valued reward is the group's target, and they will attain the established goal to achieve the reward. The overlay of goals is seen frequently in nursing courses. Students are given a goal by a teacher (teacher is a leader in this situation). The group (students) do not think the goal, which may be the learning of a particular concept or the production of a paper as evidence that a concept has been mastered, is important or of value. If the reward for learning the concept and producing the paper is an "A" (which is one quarter of the total grade for the course) and if the student's goal is an "A" in the course, then he is willing to achieve the teacher's goal (something the student does not value) to attain the reward or the real goal. Goal overlay is a common phenomenon.

PREDICTIVE PRINCIPLE: *Continuity of competent leadership facilitates the efficiency of communication process.*

Continuity, with reference to nursing care, means provision for daily, uninterrupted service for a prescribed period of time. To assure continuity there is a related chain of communications, events, and responsibilities that is unbroken. When a link in this chain becomes weak or is severed, discontinuity probability increases in proportion to the number of persons involved. Hence the thrust toward a return to the concept of primary care where those persons who are most concerned and involved in health care services are in communicative contact.

This necessitates adequate coverage for days off, illness, vacations, and leaves if communications are to be maintained at the desired level of operation. The leader hopes to select a replacement who is skilled in nursing, familiar with client or agency policies and procedures, has the ability to work well with others, and who has the potential to guide the client or group members in the achievement of their purposes.

Having the opportunity to experience firsthand the kind of group process in operation helps the alternate or associate leader to carry on the pattern of activity established by the primary leader and also provides a basis for joint evaluation of the process by both leaders.

It becomes evident that the above staffing formula is inadequate when prolonged absences occur. If provision is made for covering for vacation, illnesses, attendance at workshops, and leaves for other purposes, there will have to be additional personnel added for the purpose of orientation. It is well for the new nurse to become familiar with the overall plan of nursing care, to assess potential client(s) needs, and then to assign him for individual orientation into group processes within the work setting.

The importance of having a second person qualified to assume a managerial role is determined by the length of absence of the regular member. Leadership is not always dependent on the physical presence of the leader. If the individual or group understands its direction and its behavioral habits are established, basic functions can take place under minimal direction. If the time involved is extensive, it is mandatory that a prepared person fill the vacant position.

Having someone ready to take over during absences is important, but there are other benefits of having an associate. The process of teaching and preparing others for leadership helps the teacher to learn. The teacher may get a clearer picture of the job in the process of explaining it, will learn more about the abilities of the client or care givers, and will gain increased insight into the group processes involved.

The sense of cohesiveness built up in the members when management is shared results in a much more reliable process. Each person clarifies his role and his relationship to others. There is a reinforcement of the knowledge and a sense of accomplishment in seeing that plans run smoothly.

PREDICTIVE PRINCIPLE: *Characteristics of client and nurse-leader determine the type of communications that will evolve.*

Practice of nursing is gradually shifting its focus from that which is essentially curative and restorative, generally acute and chronic in nature, and practiced in hospitals or in patient facilities to the promotion of health maintenance and disease prevention. This latter practice is normally a continuum process and is increasingly becoming a part of community or emergent institutional programs. Hence the consumer of nursing services is being looked upon not as a "patient" but as a "client" who may initiate and participate in the provision of his own health care. This procedural shift from the client's passive to active role influences attitudes and behaviors concerned with communication.

The average consumer has increasing access to health care geographically and economically. Contemporary hospitals and similar agencies are often overcrowded and unable to provide for all the clients seeking admission. There is also the economic problem faced by those seeking health care who are unable to finance the higher cost of institutionalized service. Subsequently, there is a shift in the role of the nurse-leader from hospitals and other institutions to outpatient health care. This requires a varied technique of communications, for the nurse-leader must be acquainted with many types of facilities that offer health treatment in various locales. These range from national, state, and regional facilities to those provided by local communities, churches, and other groups interested in fostering health improvement among all strata of society. These health programs incorporate maintenance, curative, restorative, and rehabilitative services for the various types of health needs such as physical, mental, family planning, mother-child relationships, health supervision, teaching, and counseling.

Despite how or where client and nurse begin their relationship or contractual agreement, the nursing process involves an integral partnership in planning and implementing problem-oriented care. But members desire to feel secure in the knowledge that their leader is in control of the situation and has ability judiciously to assess, implement, and evaluate nursing services. The nurse-leader recognizes he is ultimately accountable to the independent client or to institutional management.

In settings where group work is in progress the leader makes it known that democratic procedure will be practiced wherever possible but that all members' responses are dependent on circumstances. The member is assured that a high degree of consistency of action is expected from both member and leader.

In a setting where patient care is the major focus, the leader will initiate action for the giving of care with the participants. The next step will be to clarify with the client or other care givers any issue not understood about the delegation of tasks and to develop a plan for procedure with the workers. The leader will assist the members as needed and will make expert information available when necessary. The leader will keep the attention on the goals established and will evaluate with the participants the quality of work done.

The successful leader will work to keep interpersonal relationships at a level where group effort can be productive and will encourage members to be cooperatively interdependent. With this type of leadership it is probable that a process will evolve in which there will be increased member participation, more rapid decision making, more achievement pressures within the group to accomplish its purposes, more effective communication, and better productivity.

REINFORCEMENT AND FEEDBACK

In human relationships some form of reinforcement, positive or negative, is communicated. The effective leader will use reinforcement as a means to increase each participant's identification with and effort toward individual or group goals. According to Professor B. F. Skinner of Harvard, reward, not punishment, is the most effective force for shaping human behavior. Positive reinforcement may be food, money, praise, a kiss, a smile, a fleeting nod of approval. More significant, however, is that positive feedback may consist of eliciting a right answer and knowing it is correct, or working out a problem to one's satisfaction, mastering a skill, or finding new beauty and order in words, music, and art. Every culture and subculture, all institutions such as hospitals and health agencies, and every home has its own methodology, acknowledged or unacknowledged, of employing rewards and punishments. Studies have shown, however, that in many cases direction of various group processes has relied on punishment or the threat of punishment to control subordinates and other members of the group. Or, they use ineffective forms of positive reinforcement, that is, those not in keeping with the value system, for participating. These practices ignore the most effective forms of positive reinforcement.

PREDICTIVE PRINCIPLE: *Integrative positive reinforcement increases individual identification with group goals and the participation level of the individual.*

Since the mid-1950s Ned Flanders, Edmund Amidon, John Hough, and others have been experimenting with a system to measure verbal and nonverbal group interaction styles called *interaction analysis.* A significant aspect of this analysis scheme is to measure the group leader's or instructor's ability to reinforce verbally the participants' behavior to get the members to initiate positive action toward group goals and increase retention level of the participants. *Integrative behavior influences* of the instructor or group leader are (1) accepts feelings of participants, (2) praises or encourages participation, (3) accepts or uses ideas of participants, and (4) asks questions of participants. *Directive behavior influences* are (1) lectures to the group, (2) gives directions to individuals or the group, and (3) criticizes or justifies authority.

Leaders and instructors who are more indirect are described as having integrative patterns, and those group leaders and instructors who are directive display more dominative patterns. The integrative leader is one who accepts, clarifies, and supports participants' ideas and feelings and who praises, encourages, and stimulates participation in the decision-making process. Directive or dominative leaders, on the other hand, tend to focus on introspective ideas and knowledge, give many directions and orders, criticize participants, and are concerned with justifying their own position and authority. Other studies have replicated the described analysis system indicating that the more integrative the leader (or the more he uses positive reinforcement), the higher the identification by group participants in achieving group goals. Instruments have been devised to measure group participants' retention of substance in group sessions, and again it was discovered, the greater the positive reinforcement, the greater the retention.

A direct positive relationship exists between the group leader's ability to reinforce the group members' supportive interaction and individual initiative in achieving group goals. There is a statistically significant positive relationship between a group leader's ability to reinforce group participants and the frequency of group members' support and reinforcement of each other. This is especially true in cases where the group leader uses more integrative positive reinforcement of group participants. The more a nurse-leader accepts, clarifies, or uses the ideas of a member, the more that member will tend to participate in the group process and positively support other members by recognizing, clarifying, and accepting their ideas and input. The behavior of nonparticipating members and isolates in a group may be changed from passive to active if the nurse-leader provides sufficient positive reinforcement to the group, since the more active participants will then in turn desire to support these less active group members through questions, encouragement, or praise or, in general, communicate a feeling of acceptance.

PREDICTIVE PRINCIPLE: *Perceiving negative feedback enables group members to become aware of others' responses to them and of their effects on the group and to evaluate goal attainment and to modify behavior accordingly.*

Negative feedback is reinforcing in that it provides individuals with important information about what is not occurring that should be, or what is happening that should not be. It enables individuals to know how they affect others in displeasing or unacceptable ways. Negative feedback is the counterpart of positive feedback, and both are important reinforcing factors. If a care giver is not contributing to group goals, nor participating in collaborative efforts, or has undesirable behaviors, it is more important for that individual to know what those noncontributory behaviors are than to proceed erroneously in ignorance.

Negative feedback is difficult for most people in that they wish to be liked, to behave appropriately, to contribute to group effort, and to be a working interdependent member. Negative feedback is often interpreted as not fulfilling their positive self-image. The pain of receiving negative input is partially offset by the knowledge of the "caring" behind the critique. Negative feedback is difficult for most people to give and therefore is avoided. Inherent in any feedback, negative or positive, there should be an attitude of "I care about you and your contribution to this group."

PREDICTIVE PRINCIPLE: *The dependent, interdependent and/or independent natures of relationships affect the structure of the communication process.*

Dependence in relationships takes three forms: (1) dependence of one member upon another for guidelines and support of action, (2) interdependence, where trust is transferred to total membership and responsibility is shared, and (3) independence, where a member engages in the activity that enhances his own development and benefits the client or group.

In communicating, members seek to achieve some balance of dependence, interdependence, and independence within its structure, according to individual needs. Successful exercise of authority requires not only a recognized dependence on the part of the members or the leader but also a reciprocal and acknowledged recognition of the leader's dependence on the members. This results in greater mutual confidence between leader and members.

Some people find comfort in maintaining close dependent relationships. These individuals usually attempt to seek constant direction and reassurance from others and may become attached to another person or persons as well. Often dependency is shown by what people do not do; it makes them unwilling to take chances, to exert extra effort, to use their imagination, or to display initiative. They achieve a degree of security without risk.

It is unwise to attempt to move the insecure individual beyond that which he is capable of accomplishing. In addition, before remedial action is taken, one must be certain that the dependent one's abilities have been weighed carefully and that he is considered to be capable of progressing beyond his present state of immaturity.

Interdependence is a reciprocal reliance between leader and participants, helping to keep the members in constant communication. In a cooperative environment, whenever one member performs a beneficial act, he simultaneously benefits all others.

An example of interdependence in action can be illustrated by the following:

A vocational nurse observed that Mr. Cable, a 68-year-old man hospitalized for treatment of a fractured femur, was developing a reddened area on his coccyx. He resisted lying on his side and disliked the treatment of massage. In checking his record the licensed vocational nurse (LVN) noted that no reference was made to this problem. After discussing the matter with the nurse leader, the LVN obtained an air mattress for Mr. Cable and then began to make plans with him for exercises he could do to increase his circulation. She followed through by recording the care plan on the nurses' notes.

This worker initiated preventive measures that would prove physically beneficial to the patient (possibly saving him a long hospitalization) and would help other care givers by affording them the satisfaction of knowing they had participated in problem-oriented care and had possibly averted many hours of unnecessary nursing care.

A state of dependence among members can foster characteristics detrimental to group goals. The nurses who gradually develop habits of coming to work a few minutes late ("nobody gets here on time; why should I?") or who become satisfied to administer minimal care so they can take extended coffee breaks are examples. Each person depends on the other to keep the "status quo," and there is resentment if moves are made to alter procedure.

The alert manager of a related group will know when conditions warrant group decision to solve the problem. The leader who can create conditions of interdependence where members perceive they will satisfy their needs by working toward common objectives will have gained the ultimate in communication process.

PREDICTIVE PRINCIPLE: *The interdependent collaborating group facilitates group goal accomplishment.*

Group participation in coordinating activities is a natural by-product of a democratic managerial philosophy. If nursing membership can facilitate coordination at the operative level, the entire organization is benefited.

Ingredients for group success in devising plans for cooperative effort include (1) a willingness on the part of all members to participate in the planning, (2) a sharing of common purposes, (3) careful communications, and (4) adherence to authority of the employing person or organization.

It has been established that responsibility for group action is vested in the leader, but this does not imply that authority must be given to a single individual. Within these guidelines, members are free to explore processes through which care can be administered to a number of patients.

Interdependent activity operates on the basic premise that group decision has the power to produce changes in individual behavior to the end that more work will be accomplished collectively than would be if attempted on an individual basis. This concept is currently being reviewed in the light of newer developments.

Cooperation is dependent upon routine relationships developed and practiced over a long period of time. It is reliant upon codes of behavior whereby people work together in a group without conscious choice of whether they will or will not cooperate. Cooperation demands a certain stability in the ways of the group. In nursing, this stability is often in jeopardy because of the fluctuating staffing pattern. In agencies where round-the-clock coverage is necessary, membership is relatively unstable and ways must be found to overcome the odds.

Group consensus presents an element of danger. The pressure of conformity, the urge to become like every other member, and the fear of the consequences if group norms are not adhered to may make a member function in a manner contrary to his value system:

> The new nurses' aide is told by her peer, "I know they told you in in-service to bathe everybody everyday, but let's face it!—we don't have that kind of time. You do up the worst ones and take care of the rest the best way you can. I give patients assigned to me a bath about two times a week. I do the best I can and report 'bath given' when we sign off."

The new aide is in a dilemma. She needs the job and wants to give good nursing care but feels pressure from all sides. She is caught in a power struggle between the tug of the stated authority figures who set the standards and the pull of one member to digress from the rules. The solution rests in the leader's ability to recognize that a power struggle exists and to deal with the situation openly. The leader can help the members face the problem by stating directly, "I notice there is a conflict between policy and practice. I need to know more about the situation. What is really going on? What caused this to happen? How do you feel about the situation?"

In all probability, group process will lead to the formation of a work structure that will resolve the conflict. The leader can ask the group how they believe priorities can best be established to ensure the administration of good care without rigidity. Possible alternatives are as follows:

1. Provide personal hygiene for every patient daily.
2. Everyday, bathe those patients having fevers, diaphoresis, or incontinence.
3. Bathe geriatric patients every other day (unless in category 2).
4. Establish round-the-clock activities (bathe some patients in evening; unresponsive patients at night).

Through interdependent action the leader has helped turn a negative situation into one that can prove highly beneficial to all concerned.

Positive interteam relationships facilitate cohesiveness and achievement of goals with speed and efficiency. Independent activity has a definite place in group activities. When a member experiences a feeling of security in his ability and in his relationships with others, he will begin to seek ways of utilizing his capacities and skills more fully. This active search is constructive and should be nurtured. The process of allowing independence among membership is a delicate one. A willingness to assume authority for special tasks does not ensure success. Self-development must have reached a level where the individual can move into the desired role with ability to achieve. Independence can be fostered by giving additional tasks gradually, so the worker is not suddenly made insecure by too great a load but can exercise his authority with discretion.

Independent action within nursing takes several routes, ranging from physical activity to mental exercise. The nurse might have sanction to manage and complete a complex assignment (for example, primary care), to take responsibility for reorganizing the medicine or treatment room, or to devise a new way to administer a treatment. The individual expresses his ideas and contributes his suggestions on matters that involve the client, himself, and group operation. Participation of this kind leads to member satisfaction in knowing that individual efforts have been recognized and that opinions and ideas are given consideration in the search for increased effectiveness and efficiency and solutions to problem-oriented nursing care.

PREDICTIVE PRINCIPLE: *Continuing reference and clarification of goals enhance the ability to attain those goals.*

Goals will seem more attainable to the participant if the nurse-leader provides opportunity for membership input. Often the group leader will assume that the preestablished goals are clear, relevant, adequate, and interesting to the extent that mere exposure will motivate the participant to achieve the goals. Empirical data suggest that increased group participation in clarifying individual and group goals is important to continual goal-directed effort; tangential activities are fewer, and group effort more consistent.

There are several methods the nurse-leader may use to determine whether the participant has perceived the relevancy of the purpose and accepts its value. The group leader should provide various types of incentives or positive reinforcement to encourage discussion of goals, values, and motivation. For example, when a client is motivated to learn or participate in the administration of isolation technique, his extrinsic and intrinsic rewards may be in achieving self-protection and in demonstrating to himself and his nurse-teacher that a complex skill has been mastered. At times the reward may be so far removed from the goal that the participant does not see the relationship. For instance, the client may see no relationship between hand washing and contamination and thus may fail to become interested in the project.

COMMUNICATION STRATEGIES

Strategies are heuristic devices or tools useful for accomplishing goals. A mechanic is equipped with a huge number of instruments, and each is designed to achieve a specific purpose and has a definite use. Some of his tools are helpful for a wider number of "jobs" than others. For instance, a spark plug wrench is singularly designed for removing and replacing spark plugs and is not applicable to many other functions, while screwdrivers, pliers, crescent wrenches, and other more nonspecific tools have a wider use for a variety of mechanical problems. Strategies are similar. The direct question, as a strategy, is useful for reviewing specific answers and definite information but may not be helpful in eliciting discussions about problems important to the group but not included in the question. Nondirective techniques may enable the client to follow his own needs and line of thought but may not provide the nurse-leader with information that is vital to a nursing diagnosis and prescription.

There are literally thousands of communication heuristics—communication group laboratory experiences, books, and courses—each filled with devices that enable individuals and groups to communicate more advantageously. This discussion does not attempt to cover even a representative number. A few devices are chosen as examples.

PREDICTIVE PRINCIPLE: *The type of communications at work in a group predicts member perception and resultant action.*

PREDICTIVE PRINCIPLE: *Congruent behavioral and verbal messages promote clear communication.*

Methods of communication employed by participants are important, for getting ideas across clearly is essential to accomplishing purposes. Improvement in communications depends on daily work among all participants to keep lines free.

Persons who know what is expected of them, who learn about changes before they take place, who feel free to clarify vague messages, and who check out unknown factors will perceive their roles in the best light and will work with heightened interest and enthusiasm.

Careful use of physical behavior and verbal delivery is an effective means of increasing communication with others. Effective communication depends upon all participants understanding the meaning of the encounter. Without effective communications, functions, and messages, a group becomes merely a collection of individuals working in close proximity and engaged in ill-defined tasks.

Communication takes many forms and is expressed either verbally or nonverbally. *Verbal communications* consists of words written or spoken to convey a message. When information or instructions are being given, it is important that the message be delivered clearly, explicitly, and to the point. When the meaning of a directive is clear, it can be carried out with ease. For example, instructions to "rotate turning the patient from back to right side, to face, to left every hour during the day" are far more likely to be carried out than instructions to "see that the patient is turned today." Nursing jargon is another facet to consider. It should be used only if the listener understands the terminology. Experienced care givers and clients might be quite comfortable hearing about "b.i.d.," "specs.," and "p.o.," but the novice may be filled with consternation at hearing even a single term.

On the other hand, most of communications is not instruction giving but collaborating for problem solving. This requires techniques that will elicit remarks and responses, provide feedback, clarify, generate ideas, help evaluate alternatives, and ultimately make goal-fulfilling choices.

Feedback is essential in the development of member's desirable qualities. In this way members can check their conception of self with how members perceive them. Confirmation of one's self-image can be pleasant and rewarding, while rejection of one's behavior may be unpleasant and even painful. Behavior can be altered if the group helps, sustains, and supports the individual through this difficult process. If the process is successful, both the individual and group members are improved by the experience.

Listening is another important behavior in the communication process, for it can convey various patterns to the speaker and other group members. The manner in which a person listens often indicates attitudes ranging from rejection or indifference to keen interest. When one listens, he makes a conscious effort to hear. The degree of attention given to the words spoken determines, to a large degree, the responses made and satisfactory performance in the work scene.

Clarifying purposes or information may be necessary before a participant can continue to follow the message. But participants must feel they can interrupt one another when necessary, or they are likely to remain silent and uninformed. Feedback can be necessary when there is a lack of comprehension. Remarks such as "Would you like to review that again?" or "Please give that back to me— I'm not sure we covered all the important points" will indicate by response that the intent of the message has been understood.

Those who spend a major share of their time in communicating ideas or feelings should deliberately work to acquire ease in establishing contact with others to enhance communicative effort, particularly in such close settings.

Congruence between actions and words is essential to clear perception and interpretations. If an individual says he understands but continues to look puzzled, the communicant has a conflict in verbal and behavioral message that he then must validate to determine which message is correct. The strategy for this is clarification. The operationalization of that strategy may take several forms:

1. *Check out:* Do you really understand?
2. *Playback:* Tell me what you heard me say.
3. *Feedback:* You look puzzled. Are you?
4. *Repeat:* Can I go through that in a different way? I may not have been very clear that time.

A strategy is a plan for action; an operation is how that plan is put into effect. The above illustrates how the plan clarification might be operationalized in four ways.

PREDICTIVE PRINCIPLE: *Threat and resulting anxiety, unless resolved, can inhibit individual and group functioning.*

Threat is a heuristic device that usually results in anxiety and can have detrimental effects on individuals and groups. Anxiety appears when there is uncertainty regarding some event or series of happenings. The tension may be expressed internally, or the feeling may be communicated to all those who have contact with the disturbed person. Anxiety can be relieved constructively through exploration of the cause of the worry with appropriate follow-up by the nurse-leader.

The effect that anxiety can have upon a care giver is illustrated through the following incident:

> John, an orderly, was evidencing anxiety feelings that were affecting his ability to function adequately. It was nearly time for his six-month evaluation when he would be informed whether he would be placed on permanent status or would be asked to leave. He was a medical student and depended on the job for his income. Besides, he liked the work and all the members of the group. When the nurse-leader gave him his three-month evaluation, he was told that his work was "O.K." but that he needed to improve. Nothing specific was mentioned. Since that time, he found himself increasingly unable to concentrate on the job.
>
> The nurse-leader confronted the orderly with his erratic behavior. Through discussion it was revealed that John was "worried sick" and because he had failed to hear any positive feedback except for an occasional noncommittal remark from his leader he

attempted to elicit some evaluation of his work from the leader. Together they discovered he had used such nonspecific means with the leader as, "Mr. Cox sure looked better today after I finished with him, don't you think?" "I categorized all the traction equipment this afternoon. It should be easier for everybody to find what they need from now on, right?"

The two members worked through the problem by analyzing the specific incidents and recognizing when feelings of anxiety were generated. The leader recognized the lack of specificity in the three-month evaluation and failure to provide structure for follow-up. John was negligent in failing to seek more direct ways for ascertaining his progress from the leader.

Another manifestation of interference with communication process is the introduction of threatening stimuli. Threat occurs where impending danger is made known by word or action. The term is applied alike to important and trivial matters. When the member becomes aware of the threat, he concentrates on ways to handle the problem. In interrelationships, threats are conveyed both through conscious and subconscious means. If, for example, two members of a group distrust one another, threatening actions expressive of their feelings will be manifested in both overt and covert ways. Innuendos, verbal exchanges, and failure to assist one another are examples. These actions have a deleterious impact upon efforts. Threats can also exert positive influence by serving as strong motivators to action. The group, for example, that is presented with a challenge for which it feels ill-prepared can offset the threat of failure by mobilizing forces to obtain the tools that will enable its members to accomplish the charge.

A group may be given the opportunity to manage the treatment room serving the nursing area. The members consider this an honor. They will have the privilege of engaging in a diversity of activities that will be interesting and will increase their knowledge and skills. Some element of threat enters in, however, for there are treatments administered about which the group knows very little. For example, they may be required to assist with a proctoscopic examination or change a complex surgical dressing. What would they do if these treatments were scheduled?

The members can handle the threat of failure by (1) resolving to accept the desired assignment, (2) requesting from management time and provision to prepare for the new role, and (3) systematically arranging for all members to become familiar and proficient with the operation.

Resistive behavior is another negative force that can deter the communication process. The apprehension of not wanting certain things to take place can evoke resistive responses in clients or group members. The inspection process may create feelings of resentment. The client or care giver may ask, "Why should I be checked on? I'm capable of completing an assignment." Opposition may also take the form of reluctance or failure to accept assignment, hostility, rigidity of action, regression, or absence.

It is vital to open communications that factors causing the resistance be identified and that attempts be made to bring about some change. The strength of resistance exerted by a member is proportionate to the degree of incompatibility the individual feels to the existing situation. The following is an example of the resistive way one member coped with feelings of incompatibility with the demands of the work situation.

> The nurse-leader was troubled by the resistive behavior of one of the nurses' aides. The aide had been a contributing member for three years when she took a year's leave of absence. Upon her return to the work group, the nurses' aide seemed to be a different person. She would leave the work area for long periods of time, would fail to answer the signal lights of the patients who were her direct responsibility, and resented any implication that she was not doing her job.

> Through investigation, the leader learned that after her return, the nurses' aide found the group had grown in its complexity of assignment beyond her level of competency. The members were now caring for neurologic patients who were acutely ill. She did not understand the implications for nursing care and believed she was now a liability to the group. This realization left the aide feeling incapable of coping with the situation. Until this time she had been able to keep up with the group commitments; she resolved her problem through retreat.

This is clearly a situation for remedial action. The aide can be helped to communicate her need and can be guided into situations that will bring her in line with current knowledge and practice.

Other forces that cause disruption and conflict are excessive competitiveness, jealousy, admission of new clients and care givers, and change of leaders. Any of these can interrupt the communication process and must be reckoned with as they arise.

Examples have been offered of what can be done in given situations when principles inherent to effective communications are utilized. Some leaders may be convinced that other approaches would be more effective. The belief may be held that resolution of negative feelings lies in the establishment of a more autocratic system. Proponents of this philosophy hope that by "tightening the ropes" the offending member will come into line. Possible devices could include requiring the member to engage in an excessive number of menial tasks, subjecting him to a verbal spanking, or stripping him of his former standing in the group.

While punitive measures might get results temporarily, participants pay a high price for such action. The membership is likely to experience much absenteeism, turnover in personnel, many grievances, and a general collapse of morale that will be reflected in the quality of care administered to the clients.

PREDICTIVE PRINCIPLE: *Questions and discussion geared to second and third level theories promote cognition that is more useful in nursing activities than questions and discussion geared to first and second level theories.*

Studies have shown that more than 80% of the verbal exchange in group process is initiated with a question. Traditionally, questions are used to determine what has been learned or the status of one's thinking. Most questions posed by group leaders or instructors are asked so that the response and thinking of the respondent is at first two levels of theory and require only memory or recall. There is, then, a wide range in the quality of questions. The effective leader will use questions geared to levels III and IV of theory discussed in Chapter 1, which call for prediction or prescription. Responses to these levels of inquiry require synthesis, imagination, and creativity and encourage varying forms of problem-oriented thinking.

In developing a questioning strategy the leader will realize that (1) questioning behavior helps to increase group interaction and establish feedback, (2) questions are used to assist participants' share, (3) questions are employed to lead the participant step by step to think about experiences, and (4) questions are means of sampling respondents' understanding of or ability to make application of concepts.

The skilled leader tends to have other techniques at his disposal to accomplish the goals itemized above. Statements that elicit remarks is one way; examples of these "eliciting remarks" are "Please tell me about . . . ," or "Help me to understand. . . ."

Bloom's taxonomy* classifies thinking into the following categories, which may be used in the formulation of higher and lower order questions:

1. *Memory*—recall or recognition of information
2. *Translation*—change of information into symbolic form or language
3. *Interpretation*—relationships among facts, generalizations, definitions, values, and skills
4. *Application*—solving a lifelike problem that requires the identification of the issue and the selection and use of appropriate generalizations and skills
5. *Analysis*—solving a problem in the light of conscious knowledge of the parts and forms of thinking
6. *Synthesis*—solving a problem that requires original creative thinking
7. *Evaluation*—making a judgement of good or bad, right or wrong, according to designated standards

John Gallagher and Mary Aschner† developed a system that classifies questions into four categories:

1. *Recall-descriptive*—narrow questions calling for specific facts, information or descriptions, to be presented by rote. Participants are asked only to give a response, not to do anything with it. Answers to these questions require only the lowest intellectual level.
2. *Convergent-explanation*—calling for the analysis and integration of given or remembered data. Problem solving and reasoning are often involved in this category. The answers may be predictable, but the task requires application of two or more recall items.
3. *Divergent-expansion*—calling for answers that are creative and imaginative and not empirically provable. Many different answers may be correct and acceptable.
4. *Value-evaluative*—dealing with judgment, value, and choice. The participant states his preference based upon individual values and standards.

---

*Bloom, B. S.: Taxonomy of educational objectives: the classification of educational goals. Handbook I. Cognitive domain, New York, 1956, David McKay Co., pp. 201-207.
†Gallagher, J., and Aschner, M.: A preliminary report on an analysis of classroom interaction. The Merrill Palmer quarterly of behavior and development **9**:3, 1963.

Table 1. A comparison of Dickoff, James, and Wiedenbach's four levels of theories with the theories of Bloom, and Gallagher and Aschner

DICKOFF, JAMES, AND WIEDENBACH	BLOOM	GALLAGHER AND ASCHNER
LEVEL I. Factor isolating	1. Memory recall or recognition of information	1. Recall-descriptive (specific facts)
LEVEL II. Factor relating	2. Translation or change of information into symbolic form or language 3. Interpretation or the establishment of relationships among facts, generalizations, definitions, values, and skills	
LEVEL III. Situation relating (predictive and inhibiting theories) LEVEL IV. Situation producing (prescriptive theories)	4. Analysis 5. Synthesis 6. Application 7. Evaluation	2. Convergent explanation 3. Divergent expansion 4. Value-evaluative

Both Bloom's and Gallagher and Aschner's works coincide with the four levels of theories described by Dickoff, James, and Wiedenbach, as discussed in the first chapter on theoretical framework. Table 1 indicates the correlation and provides a basis for formulation of questions and discussions.

Levels I and II, factor-isolating and factor-relating theories as adopted in this text, correspond to Bloom's first three items in his taxonomy. They are memory recall or recognition of information; translation or change of information into symbolic form or language; and interpretation or the establishment of relationships among facts, generalizations, definitions, values, and skills. Only one of Gallagher and Aschner's four categories of questions corresponds to the first two levels of theory proposed in this text. They term this level 1 or recall-descriptive. These refer to narrow questions that ask for specific facts.

Level III, situation-relating theories, which are predictive principles called predictive and inhibiting theories, and level IV, situation-producing or prescriptive theories, correspond closely to Blooms's last four groupings: (4) analysis, (5) synthesis, (6) application, and (7) evaluation, and to Gallagher and Aschner's number 2, 3, and 4 categories—convergent explanation, divergent expansion, and value-evaluative questions, respectively.

Productive groups soon learn the value of third and fourth level discussions and concentrate remarks on those two levels. The payoff for the leader and the group is more efficient and valid problem solving.

PREDICTIVE PRINCIPLE: *Use of simulation processes facilitates decision making and provides efficient means for learning problem-solving methods in a nonthreatening and safe environment.*

Simulation, as used in this discussion, affords the participant opportunity to elicit various response patterns to a set of circumstances, the content of which is comparable to that found in a real-life situation. Thus the member attains particular knowledge, understandings, or skills while being confronted with life-like situations; also he is required to apply these learnings in constructing a response. The manner in which he responds becomes a measure of the participant's grasp of the original learnings and an indicator of his abilities in reality situations.

Simulation is useful to develop decision-making skills (see Chapter 1). Since it is a structured, programmed method, feedback can be built into this format, which enables the participant to benefit from the experience in one of two ways: (1) he may observe if the course of action embarked on resulted in a desired payoff, which improved understanding of the problem-solving process. If this is so, then wise action is reinforced by the simulation. (2) Conversely, if the feedback shows the procedure resulted in ineffective decision making, he will then resort to alternative steps that lead to desirable results. One advantage of simulation is that the participant can be part of the audience and can see the whole of the circumstances in a nonthreatening and safe environment.

Participation builds a high degree of motivation and gives purpose to learning. A major benefit of using the simulation process is that more members of a group are immediately and actively involved in problem solving or decision making. Because of increased insight, changes in behavior are more rapidly facilitated. Simulation also supplies a number of contingencies that may often be encountered in the nursing arena and may not be experienced in the clinical work setting.

A further advantage of the simulation strategy is the acquisition of particular skills and knowledge. In life, normally a time lag occurs between making a decision and receiving information about the effects of the decision; there is also the possibility of making costly mistakes. Simulation provides a laboratory where experience can be gained and mistakes made. It also accelerates training and shows the effects of decisions quickly.

If properly structured, simulation will make it necessary for the participants to envision the whole of the problem: to be certain of their observations and facts, to collect, evaluate, and analyze the available information, and to develop prescriptions for nursing action. Another advantage is that alternative actions for a given circumstance can be identified and explored. During the post-simulation stage, reflection, interpretation, and discussion are often needed for final synthesizing and evaluating.

GOAL SETTING, ACHIEVEMENT, AND EVALUATION

Goal setting, prescribing nursing actions, and evaluating progress are key nursing responsibilities requiring a network of communication. Determining goals for effective nursing leadership depends on an accurate assessment of what comprises effectual management for the work situation. The goal setting individual or group must know professional standards for nursing care, be cognizant of policies and expectations for the nurse leader by the client or employer, be familiar with the work environment (physical setting, design for administration of nursing services, personnel, lines of authority), and be aware of needs and wishes of the clients who are served. Since democratic groups are facilitated by leaders to set their own goals, this task is a shared one.

Further, the nurse-leader helps goals to be communicated in meaningful terms, recognizing that (1) behavior implies active participation, (2) the learning procedure consists of acts that require a change in behavior, (3) persons respond more quickly if they assist in establishing their own goals for learning, and (4) the committed individual is motivated to achieve optimal levels of performance.

The effective nurse-leader develops skills in awareness of problems, formulation of goals, appropriate activities, methods of evaluation, and in sharing this process with involved participants in establishing aims and devising activities for their accomplishment. With this leadership, efforts are more effective, quality of care is improved, job satisfaction is increased, and costs are reduced.

PREDICTIVE PRINCIPLE: *Preassessment of individual and group knowledges, skills, and expectations establishes base-line data for measurement of progress or change.*

The primary purpose of the preassessment process is to determine what the individual or group brings to the nursing arena in terms of prerequisite knowledge for nursing activity. Planning nursing prescriptions without first making an assessment of participant characteristics is akin to prescribing medicine without first diagnosing the patient. If individuals from the least to the most skilled are to be given adequate opportunity to progress and achieve, the nurse-leader needs to assist members in determining their status and the procedural method. As the nurse-leader gains information regarding each client and care giver or related person, strategies can be developed and plans made for reducing the discrepancy between what the participant is able to achieve now (at the point of preassessment) and what he can be expected to accomplish within a prescribed period of time.

It is vital to ascertain what the participants have learned, what skill levels they have achieved, and what characteristics they possess in order to avoid lessening interest and motivation through unnecessary repetition and consequent boredom. Through preassessment process, the nurse-leader can develop base-line data for the measurement of progress or change that result from the members' experiences and instruction in nursing practice. For example, the leader determines from preassessment that a nurse is unable to take a maternal-child health history at the beginning of the work experience. If at the end of the designated learning activity the member is able to make a complete nursing assessment, success has been attained. Without preassessment it would be difficult, if not impossible for the leader to ascertain how or when learning and change in behavior occurred.

While it would seem impossible for the nurse-leader to be totally aware of the interests, concerns, and expectations of each entering client and nurse-participant, goals are achieved with greater efficiency when the leader communicates closely with the members by preassessing, accepting, and clarifying the expectations, interests and concerns of each member. Often a client or worker enters the nursing scene expecting a certain experience, only to be disappointed, confused, and frustrated because the direction and focus is not what he expected or perceived himself as needing. The effective leader will preassess individual participant expectations and align these expectations with related activities to the extent that the care plan and environment permit.

PREDICTIVE PRINCIPLE: *Mutual understanding and agreement on goals appropriate to the client or agency ensure support for goal achievement.*

Agencies are established for specific and defined purposes. These purposes are dictated by social and community health needs and are written into charters and agency objectives. When an individual becomes an employee of an agency, he commits himself to the agency's established purposes. Agencies support activities designed to accomplish goals in keeping with the defined purposes of the agency. Support for activities outside the defined purposes is not economically feasible and dissipates the manpower necessary for the accomplishment of established agency purposes. Such purposes change when social, health, or community needs dictate alteration, either by evolution or through responses to emergency situations (civil, natural, or national disasters). Agency purposes seldom change simply because nursing care groups adopt goals not in keeping with established ends. Therefore, it behooves nursing groups to select goals appropriate to the institution to ensure its support. The following example is illustrative of the principle under discussion:

> Jimmie Bigalow, an 8-year-old boy, had been in Sundown Children's Convalescent Hospital for 18 months for convalescence from rheumatic fever with several complications when he became acutely ill with pneumonia, laryngeal edema, high fever, and severely compromised respiration. The hospital management wanted Jimmie transferred to an acute hospital immediately. The nurses had become extremely attached to Jimmie and were very concerned about his care. The nursing group volunteered to "special" Jimmie and to devote their days off to his care. They requested that the hospital secure the necessary equipment through rental or purchase and give permission to the unit to keep and care for Jimmie. The request was denied for the following reasons:
> 1. The hospital plant and equipment was designed for convalescing children.
> 2. Other patients on the unit would feel the impact of a critically ill patient through the nurses' preoccupation with Jimmie and the necessity of maintaining a quiet atmosphere.
> 3. Time off should be spent away from the job to enable full devotion to the job during scheduled work time.

An astute nurse-leader would have determined if group purposes were consistent with the agency goals and attempted to lead the membership to adoption of objectives compatible with the agency. Examples of appropriate objectives for the nursing group and goals that would have secured the support of the agency would have been (1) to prepare Jimmie for smooth transfer to another hospital and (2) to adopt measures that would decrease the separation anxiety of both patient and nursing staff.

To ensure successful cooperation of and support from the client in primary nursing or in independent care systems, it is of vital import that communication lines exist in the operation. Goals and implementation and evaluative measures must be defined by the nurse-leader in conjunction with the client or his representative, the group or agency where appropriate. Of equal significance in establishing a procedural health measure is the nurse-leader and the client. In all independent negotiations care will be exercised that the legal rights of both the consumer of health care services and the rendering person or agency be protected.

PREDICTIVE PRINCIPLE: *Circumstance and member capability determine the type of direction to be communicated.*

The types of direction most nurse-leaders are likely to give are (1) the command, (2) the request, (3) the suggestion, and (4) the call for volunteers.

A *command* is an authoritative direction or order; it is an exercise of direct authority. Commands imply set directives and structure and require little discussion. Some directions are communicated as commands because the implementation of the directives is important to safety, subsequent activities, cooperation with other departments, or the implementaion of physicians' orders.

There are times when the *request* can be used to better advantage, and so far as the worker is concerned, carries almost the same weight as a direct command. Usually the request is given in situations where the time schedule is flexible and the worker is capable of exercising judgment. An example would be, "Mrs. Blanton, when you have a chance would you investigate other ways of arranging Mrs. Sampson's personal effects so she can use them more easily. Her right arm is becoming less useful to her each day. She has indicated a desire to use her left arm more." Another form of request could be, "I wonder if you would spend some time with Mr. Berra. He feels lonely because his son and family have moved from this area." The request indicates that compliance is expected but that freedom of choice exists.

In the *suggestion* category decisions are left to the worker as to whether something will be done. Suggestions offer alternatives or choices. "If Mrs. Hill is having difficulty swallowing liquids, you might try semisolids," and "You could call the welfare department and find out what they think," are examples of suggestions. Suggestions do much to stimulate initiative and cooperation in the members for they provide opportunities for the use of independent judgment.

The *request for volunteers* is a form used occasionally in soliciting people for assignments that are beyond usual duties or are difficult or unpleasant. Assisting in another area, serving on a special committee, or assuming responsibility for reorganizing the utility room are examples of situations for which all members have a choice. Again, the leader must exercise caution not to place himself in the awkward position of having to refuse a volunteer for a job for which he feels the worker is not qualified or of having no one volunteer for a job that must be done. If the possible candidates are limited, then the call should go out only to those who are qualified to accept. For example, "I would like John, June, or Mary to take care of this; will one of you volunteer?"

There is dual responsibility (leader and member) for preventing continuous delegation of extra tasks to the same few individuals. In every group are certain workers who are more cooperative than others and who, unless protected, may be exploited.

Conversely, there is a reciprocal relationship in which the client may at times be the communicator of directions. He may determine in collaboration with the primary care giver the manner in which he desires his care or health plan to be implemented. The client may outline specific times, places, procedures, resources, and persons to fulfill his care plan.

Several rules of thumb hold firm in the giving of directions or suggestions:

1. *Do not give a choice if there is no choice.* "Would you like to help Mrs. Jones?" Implies a "no" response is acceptable. If you mean "Please help Mrs. Jones," then say so. A better alternative for giving choice yet eliciting a positive response is the question. "Would you be willing to help Mrs. Jones?" Many people who do not want to "especially" would be willing to.

2. *When offering suggestions make certain they are viewed as suggestions and not dictums.* After offering a suggestion, recommend the person get ideas from others so that he will have a wider choice of alternatives.

3. *When issuing a command or order, make it clear it is an expectation.* "Mrs. Jones' tray is here now," is a simple statement of fact and does not even imply what you want done with that tray. If you wish Mrs. Jones to have her tray while it is hot, say so, for example, "Please take Mrs. Jones her tray while it is still hot; it just arrived from the kitchen."

4. *Provide choices when choices are possible.* Even a limited amount of freedom of choice is better than no choice at all. "I'm sorry, Mrs. Lucie, you cannot save your break until this afternoon and take off early because there is a meeting that Mrs. Copty and Mrs. Gill must attend at that time, and you and I will be alone for 30 minutes. However, you can alter your schedule either Thursday or Friday—both those days are clear."

PREDICTIVE PRINCIPLE: *Opportunity to express expectations of the individual or group, when translated into meaningful terms to members, relates directly to individual identification and invites commitment of members to goal achievement.*

Goal setting and evaluation are the lifeblood of nursing effort. Goal setting gives nursing activities meaning; evaluation allows the group to measure fulfillment; success whets the appetite for more achievement and motivates the individual or group to further meaningful activity.

Whether an individual or group goal or process is sufficiently important to exert an effect on a participant's behavior depends upon the goal's relationship to the person. The possibilities of what might be expected are many. Confronted with a goal or process, the participant will be uncertain about what to expect but will seek that which has meaning to him. Perceptions and expectations are a selective process and are based on past experiences and present awareness. The participant will attend to those matters and anticipate goals and processes that have a relationship to self or to an extension of the self. Information will affect a person's behavior only to the degree to which he has discovered its personal meaning for himself.

It is important, therefore, that the nurse leader provide opportunity for the client, individual, or group member to express and clarify his initial expectations.

When the participant has opportunity to express his desires, he is more willing to accept the established goals and intended processes of the group. The more responsive the leader is to the participant's expectancies, the less his resistance to the group's intended goals or processes. The effective group leader will structure the situation so that the client or member will express and clarify individual expectations.

To achieve group commitment and resultant behavior a goal must have value and meaning. The goal must be something the members can define, put into their own experience, and accept into their own value system. The following is an example:

> Miss Lee, a young graduate, was attempting to get a group composed primarily of new nursing assistants interested in foot care for a middle-aged diabetic man. She discussed, at great length, improving circulation, proper shoes, the care of toenails and corns, and bathing and powdering the feet. The group was completely passive until an experienced aide said: "Miss Lee, are you trying to tell us that if we don't do something, Mr. Taylor's sore toe could turn black and he could lose his foot?"

The aide's translation of the objective into something that had meaning for the group and was familiar to them aroused interest and achieved commitment to the goal.

PREDICTIVE PRINCIPLE: *Realistic and valid goals promote achievement.*

Setting goals the group can achieve motivates the individual or group to success. Goal setting and record keeping by the nurse-leader produce gratifying results. With these tools, delegation becomes less difficult and the role of the nurse expands to an amazing degree. The old saying "goals just beyond reach keep one striving" is false. Goals beyond reach are self-defeating and lead to discouragement and apathy. Realistic means achievable; valid as used here means relevant to the problem. Use of the following three simple, precautionary steps enables the nurse-leader to guide the group in the selection of realistic, valid, attainable goals:

1. *Identify problems.* Descriptions are essential to problem identification. Full, detailed descriptions of the situation and feelings about the situation empower the group to accurately identify the problem.

2. *Set goals.* Accurately identified problems make it possible for the group to foresee the termination, or at least an alteration, of the problem that would make the situation more tolerable. This imagined absence or alteration of the problem becomes the goal.

EXAMPLE: The goal for a patient who has trouble with contractures is free movement with full range of motion.

Problem	*Goal*
Contractures	Free movement with full range of motion

3. *Determine ability to accomplish goals.* Determining the group's ability to accomplish the goal establishes whether the goal is realistic. Qualities necessary to the accomplishment of a stated goal would include such things as the following:

a. *Resources*—either have or can acquire the collective or individual talent, knowledge, and skill appropriate and effective for accomplishment of the goal. When each desired behavior is defined behaviorally in terms of outcome, the learner knows what is expected specifically and can then determine his capability or resources for the tasks.

b. *Time and energy*—consideration must be given to other tasks facing the group concomitantly.

c. *Commitment and will of the group.*

PREDICTIVE PRINCIPLE: *The extent of involvement of each group member determines the proficiency of the group.*

Membership in a group necessitates some degree of personal involvement. Behavior as a group member is guided mainly by the individual's perception of his needs and interests. A member who receives satisfaction from the work experience will be motivated to join inextricably with the group.

Consideration of variables that influence member involvement is essential to understanding the working of groups.

All individuals are members of several groups, any one of which may exert much more influence on the member's life than the work situation does. Family, social clubs, religious and political affiliations, and community projects are examples of group associations that involve the individual.

Membership in a group does not necessarily engage the entire person, but group proficiency requires that each member involve himself fully toward the achievement of group purposes while he is present with the group. A few dedicated persons literally live and breathe nursing and evidence little interest in outside activities. These members have much to contribute, but unless they are carefully controlled, they can dominate the group and destroy its effectiveness. The overly zealous member becomes wearisome to others and eventually creates a backlash of negative reaction that takes its toll in group productivity.

The leader can utilize the devoted member's zeal constructively by channeling some of the worker's energy into activities that can be performed on an individual basis. Keeping the ward library up-to-date is one way of providing helpful diversion. The interested member could search nursing literature and bring pertinent materials to the station for members of all teams. Another avenue for the individual deeply engrossed in the profession is serving on nursing procedure committees, policy boards, and so on. Care must be taken to ensure broad representation, but usually all who wish to do so have the opportunity to participate in these kinds of activities. There are numerous worthwhile but time-consuming tasks in committee work. The eager member can volunteer to devote as much time and effort as he desires to these responsibilities.

A problem of equal significance is the member who works eight hours a day, five days a week for a paycheck and evidences little or no interest in the endeavors of the nursing group to which he is assigned. This person must be assisted to progress from his dormant or even inhibitory stage to one of productivity, or his position as a group member will become untenable.

Possible reasons for the lack of member involvement might be that conditions in the work setting are not contributing to member satisfaction. Perhaps the staff member does not feel accepted as a necessary part of the group process. Perhaps he rarely has the opportunity to complete assigned tasks without interruption. Perhaps he does not feel secure in his ability to perform the assigned tasks (tests in management reveal a close relationship between ability and interest). On the other hand, he may not experience sufficient outlet for his abilities. It is up to group participants to discover conditions that will promote and maintain interest in their work situation to foster member involvement and to pave the way for group proficiency.

Another factor that influences the extent of involvement an individual has in a group is the degree to which the beliefs, values, and attitudes of the group conflict or agree with those of other groups to which he belongs. Conformity pressures may be exerted from both sides, thus forcing the individual to make a choice between the two. This type of conflict occurred when a community health nurse was assigned to head a team in a district that was predominantly populated by Mexican-Americans. The first three-month report revealed very little progress with the families to which she was assigned. Upon consultation with the nurse the supervisor learned the leader had been indoctrinated since childhood by both family and social groups to believe that "Mexicans are stupid and lazy, do not wish to work, and have as many children as possible in order to collect welfare."

The administrator believed the nurse could become a competent and contributing member of the staff. Accordingly, the nurse was assigned to a different district with the provision that she study Mexican-American culture through attendance of classes and participation in seminar discussions within the health department where families of Mexican heritage were reviewed. The supervisor reasoned that families could not receive help from a biased leader; therefore a change in staffing was necessary. The assignment to attend classes and seminars was based on the assumption that, with increased understanding of Mexican-American culture, the nurse would have an opportunity to examine her pre-sets and would become able to work in the first assignment.

Lack of involvement in group process may result when individual member beliefs and team goals are in conflict. Inadequate attention to the patient may be given, or possible acts of negligence may be committed when conflict exists. For example, a nurse who feels strongly that the administration of blood by transfusion is morally wrong may subconsciously (or even consciously) avoid observing the patient for signs of reaction or may neglect other important needs involved in the treatment. Another example is the group member who rejects the right of patients to take oral contraceptives. If the nurse member makes her views known to the patient, the patient receiving such medication will feel she must justify her actions to the nurse.

One primary aim of the nurse-leader is to bring all members of the group having different norms or values into a functioning relationship. Possible means include providing the group members with a role model through exemplary leadership, group discussions, individual conferences, and workshops with continuous exposure of the members to a democratic point of view.

Actions in the interest of the patient are to be fostered; if the decision is reached that the member cannot resolve his conflict and become involved in the achievement of the group's purposes, the leader will be forced to recommend his removal from the work group.

PREDICTIVE PRINCIPLE: *Group involvement in goal setting necessitates the endorsement of the agency and commitment of membership to participate in the outcome.*

Group decisions in formulating goals can have a place in employee relations but must be limited to issues that are reasonable and obtainable through the conscientious efforts of all personnel.

Like most business and industrial organizations, health agencies follow established patterns of operations. A governing board gives direction and overall guidance, the administrators furnish the physical environment and services that support the medical and nursing staff, and formulated and stated policies provide guidelines for all administrative action. Ideally, leaders of nursing groups have a part in the formulation of overall policy, but in any case, the leader is governed by the stipulations of the employing agency.

In nursing teams, formation of group goals has more the character of selecting subgoals for procedure. Group aspirations are subordinate to those objectives outlined for all nursing services. Overall goals for the agency are usually stated in general terms such as, "To provide nursing care commensurate with the standards established by the American Nurses Association," or "To treat all patients equally." It is important to recognize that while these goals may be desirable and members of the nursing group may wish to become involved in their implementation, they are too vague for specific operation. Examples of goals that imply member involvement are (1) complete a course in cardiac resuscitation, (2) develop a plan that would facilitate interaction among members, and (3) and increase care giver skill in the operation of cardiac monitors. Each of these aims can be worked through operationally and can be sucessfully accomplished according to the extent of member involvement.

With the kind of objectives just given, participants can work cooperatively to design a plan that will lead to specific realization. The latter objective could be operationally defined by the group in the following way:

GOAL: To increase care giver skill in the operation of cardiac monitors.

OPERATION:

1. Provide each member with a copy of a manual containing necessary background information.
2. Allow two weeks for individual study.
3. Set up a series of one-hour seminars with in-service director and staff in charge of the cardiac unit.
4. Arrange for practice sessions with equipment. Arrange schedule so that each member has adequate time to attend seminars and practice sessions (equal time does not necessarily have to be given to each member).
5. Have each member take test on theory and practice.
6. Plan additional seminars and practice sessions according to individual need.
7. Allow time for review periods at least once per month.

As the members become involved in planning steps to reach their goal, they will designate the persons who are to assume responsibility for implementation. Total involvement takes place throughout the process, thus committing members to the outcome.

A managerial error is made when a group is allowed to participate in decisions for which there can be no subsequent fulfillment. The following is an example:

> Mrs. Beaux, leader of a nursing team, attended a seminar on group dynamics and was particularly impressed with a series of lectures given about employees who were setting their own goals for job fulfillment. The speaker emphasized that if co-workers were given the opportunity, they could meet together to intelligently consider and then formulate goals that would be appropriate to the situation.
>
> Returning to her nursing station, Mrs. Beaux decided to practice some of the principles she had heard. She called together the five members of her team and told them that, in her opinion, the team members would be more satisfied if they decided just how much work they could accomplish in one day. She then gave the team members the opportunity to discuss and to decide among themselves as a group what their work load should be. Mrs. Beaux left the room, believing the group would doubtlessly assess their jobs and establish much higher goals for themselves than she herself would have dared propose.
>
> After the discussion period was over, the group informed Mrs. Beaux they believed they were overworked. Since they had been given the authority to establish their own work load, they would reduce the patient census on their team by two and would relinquish their responsibility for distributing fresh linens to all teams.

The weakness in the original proposal belatedly became clear to Mrs. Beaux. She had allowed individuals to participate in a decision that could not be realized, for she did not have the power to implement the proposal. She had failed to equate her naive assumption with reality and was left with a disastrous situation.

The fiasco could have been avoided had the nurse-leader consulted with the head nurse first to see if the plan was feasible and workable. Mrs. Beaux must now use the situation as a bad start toward something better. She can tell the group where the idea originated, what she thought would happen, and the situation she finds herself in now. She can discuss with the group the matter of feelings of overload in work assignment and attempt to work out a solution with them within the present structure that is mutually satisfactory to both. By this method the nurse-leader's ideas, the group's wishes, and the guidelines and policies of the institution can be blended into a constructive approach.

EFFECTIVE CONFERENCES

Conferences are necessary to the practice of nursing to give and to receive information cooperatively and collaboratively.

Grouping persons involved in accomplishing common goals for the purpose of interchange of ideas and solving problems provides a useful tool for building and maintaining mutual understanding.

Nursing conferences are not limited to providers of health services. It is now generally recognized that to attain and maintain optimum mental and physical health, if possible, all significant persons must be included in each phase of client care. Thus, in addition to members of the health team, the client, his family, and others who have an interest in the purpose of the conference are included.

A nursing conference is usually called for the purpose of finding out or deciding something. This means there is a reciprocal relationship for the exchange of information. Nurses convene conferences for a variety of purposes. These include (1) direction-giving conferences, in which the leader or client gives information and direction specific to the assignment, (2) patient-centered conferences, in which members identify problems and attempt to arrive at solutions and decide upon courses of action, (3) content conferences, in which participants assemble to acquire knowledge about a specific subject, (4) reporting conferences, in which participants give progress reports, (5) general problems conferences, in which individuals express their impressions about the work situation and try to resolve work or personnel problems, and (6) primary care conferences, in which participants collaborate for problem-oriented nursing care.

Effective communication necessitates a systematic plan for providing and maintaining contact between the leader and group and for person-to-person exchanges. Gathering groups together at specific times for clearly defined purposes will help to realize this goal.

The time for nursing conferences is usually relatively short; therefore the discussants must work for brevity and exactness. Conference style is most often informal and more conversational than formal meetings; therefore the group must be cognizant of the need to be purposeful and well organized.

The conference situation is not a "natural" one for the nurse-leader, and many are tempted to find reasons for not meeting with the entire group at one time. The leader who feels ill at ease in conducting group sessions, for example, may look for reasons to cancel meetings. The excuse may be offered, "There never seems to be a right time to get the group together—when I'm ready, they're not. I would like to have them meet all at one time, but there are just so many hours in a day!" The alternative action is to "catch them on the run" or, worse yet, to trust that the members will discover for themselves what is expected of them.

Time is an important factor, as most care givers spend the greater share of their work period attempting to meet the numerous demands placed upon them. It is true, however, that most people find time for activities they deem important and in which they feel comfortable. If one accepts the principle that effort to arrive at group consensus for nursing action cultivates positive outcomes, then time must be given to meetings where the process can take place.

The leader can become adept in the role of conference leader if effort is channeled into acquiring and applying principles of conference technique that will contribute to the realization of effective amalgamation of ideas and feelings.

All conferences have certain commonalities. Accomplishment of purpose is enhanced when members have the opportunity to meet without interruption and come prepared to participate and when behaviors enhance goal accomplishment. Another contributing factor to successful conference sessions is participant understanding of behaviors each individual uses to impart ideas or feelings to others and recognition of the effect specific actions have on the group.

PREDICTIVE PRINCIPLE: *Adequate preparation by the leader for all conferences expedites fulfillment of expectations for the conference.*

Realities of life make adequate preparation for all situations at all times impossible. Nursing is particularly susceptible to disruptions. New patients are admitted just prior to conference time; substitute staff are assigned; new procedures are introduced; emergencies occur; and friction occasionally arises among health personnel. In addition to these disruptive elements, the nurse-leaders will not necessarily have acquired competency in all phases of nursing. Deviations from the ideal, however, need not deter the nurse-leader from proceeding with preparation as current conditions allow.

Preparation for a conference will depend upon the purpose of the meeting. Instructional conferences call for imparting information to members to facilitate completion of assignments. Content and patient-centered conferences require acquisition of knowledge specific to a particular patient or subject. Reporting conferences demand that the reporter know what needs reporting; the content and shared feelings conferences depend upon group needs coupled with judicious use of interpersonal relationship skills.

PREDICTIVE PRINCIPLE: *Relieving care givers of responsibility while conference is in session allows members to proceed without interruption.*

In most clinical settings, more than one nurse or group is assigned to care for the total patient population. Leaders will want to coordinate their schedules to allow time for necessary meetings and to arrange for the care of patients assigned to them while each group is in session.

Patients should not be left unattended by nursing staff. This is especially true in acute nursing care units where lack of supervision can have serious consequences. (Intravenous fluids can accelerate or reduce in rate within seconds; patients may require assistance with bodily functions; and there is the ever present possibility of crises such as hemorrhage, shock, myocardial infarction, or cardiac arrest.)

Primary care or community health agency conference interruptions take the form of telephone calls, family disruptions, or cooperating personnel requiring the nurse's or client's time.

In structured settings a conference time schedule that considers the needs and desires of all personnel equally will prove to be the most successful. Most leaders consider the ideal time for a direction-giving conference to be as soon after the work day has started as possible. The leader will then have the opportunity to give directions to members before the group becomes involved in a multiplicity of tasks. The preferred time for the reporting conference is usually about 45 minutes before the end of the shift. This arrangement gives members the opportunity to sum up the day's progress before completing last minute details. Scheduling of content and patient-centered conferences does not usually become an issue other than to find a time when members can get together.

Nursing functions cover myriad activities. Each member has a job to do that usually must be done within a certain time limit. Some tasks demand strict compliance to a schedule. Preoperative medications and the collection of specimens illustrate this point. Other assignments, such as the administration of hygienic care, allow for a degree of flexibility. Agency and client routines must be taken into consideration. Serving of meals and provision for treatments given by those other than the nursing personnel further complicate planning care. Community health agencies usually have more freedom in scheduling activities, but regardless of setting all require careful programming.

PREDICTIVE PRINCIPLE: *Prior announcement of time, place, purpose, and duration of conferences to all concerned promotes assembly of a group well prepared and ready to focus attention on the purposes of the conference.*

The importance of holding conferences for the purpose of giving direction, coordinating activities, and evaluating progress is patent. It is equally evident that each member must know in advance when, where, how long, and for what purpose the conferences will be held.

A written schedule of meeting times is helpful. A printed format may be devised to fit any situation. Information concerning specific conferences can then be filled in easily and posted for all staff members to note. The following is a model of scheduling for an area that has three groups.

CONFERENCE	GROUP I	GROUP II	GROUP III
Direction-giving	7:30-7:50 (Daily)	8:00-8:20 (Daily)	7:30-7:50 (Daily)
Patient-centered	1:00-1:30 (Monday)	11:00-11:30 (Tuesday)	1:00-1:30 (Wednesday)
Content	1:00-1:30 (Tuesday)	11:00-11:30 (Wednesday)	1:00-1:30 (Thursday)
Report	2:15-2:35 (Daily)	1:40-2:10 (Daily)	2:15-2:35 (Daily)

When there are three groups, two can meet at one time with careful planning. The head nurse and ward secretary assist the third group in alerting the attending staff of the patients' needs. Leaders in conferences will have informed the covering nurse-leader of any specific needs that require attention during the time of the conference. When there are only two groups, scheduling is simplified. It becomes a matter of one covering for the other while they are in conference and alternating times of meetings from week to week. When only one group is involved, times for meeting together should still be scheduled, but flexibility in timing is more easily managed. In this event, coverage will be arranged on an individual basis.

All members realize there will be occasions when it is impossible to hold to the conference schedule. At such times, the situation is usually stressful, often causing the members to forget the times of meetings. If at all possible, however, the leader involved in the disruption should alert another leader to arrange for a trade in times for meetings. If the cause for the delay does not permit this step, the coordinator of nursing services must be alerted to proceed with alteration or trade in the conference schedule with the leader who is detained. Keeping one group waiting for a conference that will not be held is a waste of time, and where more than one group is involved, the time lost is proportionately increased.

When a number of people work together in close harmony, it is understandable that they will be interested in one another's lives and will take advantage of opportunities to exchange information and confidences. A few moments can be allotted for this purpose before initiating the conference or while waiting for all members to arrive. Once the meeting has begun, however, participants will need to exercise discipline to keep their attention focused on the purpose for meeting. The leader can assist the group to hold to its mark by recognizing when diversion from the appointed task has occurred and can bring the discussion back into focus by using simple phrases such as, "Can we return to . . . ," "You were saying that . . . ," or "Will you explore . . . a little further, please."

DIRECTION-GIVING CONFERENCE

Direction-giving conferences are meetings called at the beginning of a work shift for the specific purpose of communicating job assignments, delineating areas of responsibility, and imparting the information necessary for members to effectively care for patients.

PREDICTIVE PRINCIPLE: *Obtaining the most recent data available prior to conference assures the leader that imparted information is pertinent, inclusive, and accurate.*

In settings where there is round-the-clock coverage the nurse-leader will receive a progress report from the person who was previously responsible for the groups of patients either by word of mouth or via tape recorder while the off-going nurse is completing the assignment. Additional information will be needed before giving instructions to care givers. Leaders will want to check pertinent data such as preoperative orders, arrangements for tests, and so on, and to visit each patient *before* the time of the instructional conference. This will give the leader opportunity to make a personal assessment of the patient's status.

In active units, frequent attempts will be made to interrupt the time the leader has reserved for personal visits to patients. Most interruptions can be handled by delegating tasks to others. Intercommunication systems prove invaluable to the leader making rounds, allowing the nurse to keep in touch with staff and yet proceed with the intended purpose of allowing client participation in the development of his care plan and to provide for client-nurse dialogue. Informal meetings will be conducted by primary care nurses, but the need for careful preparation is not lessened. In many instances the client and his family will engage in preplanning activities by reading, experimenting with procedure, investigating resources, and so on.

PREDICTIVE PRINCIPLE: *Information to care givers and/or clients that is paced, systematic, and inclusive allows participants time to assimilate the content and provides them with information necessary to function.*

The success or failure of imparting pertinent information to an individual or a group depends on sufficient information and method of presentation. The leader must be sensitive to what information is needed and at what pace the members (client and/or care givers) are able to receive it. In a direction-giving conference, for example, members should not be avalanched with irrelevant information. They want to hear that which will be most useful to the immediate situation.

Much of the information determining routine and time of performance is a part of core information. Routine care, time for meals, procedure for obtaining or imparting information, and so on are best omitted unless there is need for review. New members will require instruction in addition to the routine information, but all members should not be subjected to the instructional part of the newcomer's orientation period.

Routine information that must be transmitted about patients, such as diet, activity, tests, and treatments, can be transcribed on care giver's work sheets by the ward clerk prior to the work period. In group conferences use of serial order on individual work sheets allows the members to know the routine, thus enabling them to increase speed and effectiveness in writing the things they have just heard.

There is a direct relationship between the requirement for information transmission and task difficulty. The amount of detail necessary in the "how" part of an order depends on how complicated the task is and how experienced the client-employee is in doing the job. For instance, there is no need to discuss nursing procedures familiar to the listener. But when the situation calls for new knowledge or skills or deeper understanding, the leader must allow time for a clear, understandable explanation.

In giving an order, a leader may neglect to explain the reason for the directive. An explanation makes it possible for the worker to use sound judgment if he has a problem, and it often helps to eliminate misunderstanding. The leader may direct an aide to "ambulate Mrs. Sheppard for five minutes every hour." The aide becomes so engrossed in the fulfillment of a heavy assignment that judgments must be made about priority. She decides to omit Mrs. Sheppard's ambulation. A simple statement to the aide at the time of the directive might have assured proper consideration when priorities were established. The leader could have explained: "Mrs. Sheppard had a vein ligation of both legs yesterday. It is very important that she walk for five minutes every hour to avoid the formation of blood clots in her legs. If one were to form and become dislodged it could travel through the bloodstream directly to her heart and cause her death."

Modern communication technology permits nurses to exchange information necessary to implement care plans in ways that provide for individual timing. Reports, directions, and communications about goal progress may be communicated via tape cassette. The oncoming staff may listen to short reports while off-going care givers continue to work with patients. Any clarification may be done by individuals at their own convenience.

PATIENT-CENTERED CONFERENCES

Patient-centered conferences are meetings in which problem-oriented care is discussed and evaluated. Patient-centered conferences are designed to help overcome the decentralization of the care of patients. The focus of attention is usually on the analysis of one patient or family situation for whom the nurse or group is caring. Patient-centered conferences provide a means whereby all participants will benefit from the experiences of a few. Where possible, the client or other signficant persons are included in the sessions and the patient is the focal point of discussion. The process is a dynamic, interactive problem-oriented approach, based upon a theoretical framework operationally defined (assessment, problem identification, formulating plans for nursing action, providing for evaluation and implementation).*

In utilizing the nursing process the leader opens the way for consideration of the needs of the whole patient—physiologic, psychologic, spiritual, social, and cultural—to acquire a rationale for nursing action and to devise ways to improve nursing care. The leader has an opportunity to guide members in recognizing individual patient or family needs and in formulating nursing principles that result in nursing prescriptions for action.

Separate meetings about patients or families, which are not in conjunction with another type of conference, allow time for discussion free from interruption. Participants will be more successful in keeping their commitment to purposes if meetings are planned at a time when the major share of the work load has been accomplished and if the conferences are well spaced. Frequency of patient-centered conferences depends on the situation. Intensive care units, for example, may not meet more than once a week, whereas an area with a slower pace might have the opportunity to meet more frequently. Thirty-minute to one-hour periods are usually sufficient for the average conference. Problem solving requires at least that much time, and little can be accomplished if the group must work under pressure.

Use of the theoretical framework, principles of teaching, learning, and leadership, will help in assisting the group to become increasingly more skilled in its ability to recognize and to solve specific problems and to make appropriate generalizations in nursing care in similar though different nursing situations.

PREDICTIVE PRINCIPLE: *Interaction of conference members on an equal basis encourages active participation and leads to usable solutions to the problem.*

Conference participants have diverse cultural, educational, and experiential backgrounds. Acceptance of the philosophy that the group together has more knowledge about a subject than any single member does, can serve to improve the productivity of the group.

---

*Bower, F. L.: The process of planning nursing care: a theoretical model, St. Louis, 1972, The C. V. Mosby Co., p. 10.

In nursing care conference situations the members make decisions by consensus or majority so that the commitment to such decisions is corporate and not vested in any one individual.

The leader must provide a nonthreatening environment if members are to feel free to share what they have done with others, engage in identification of problems, and give and receive suggestions for further action. If the leader imposes his own opinions on the group prematurely, he, in effect, negates the potential benefits that can be derived from the participation of all members.

In a nursing care conference situation the leader opens the discussion, then invites members to make contributions to the discussion freely. The leader's role is primarily one of facilitating the group work in constructing plans that will benefit a patient or family. Some conferences will require little active participation from the leader, and others will demand a larger contribution. Regardless of who offers content in the conference, each contribution should be given careful consideration. The patient or family and other significant persons may be an integral part of the process.

PREDICTIVE PRINCIPLE: *Identification of the nursing problem to be considered expedites the formulation of nursing intervention.*

The initial steps in a nursing care conference are (1) to assess the group interest and need, (2) to identify and delineate the problem, (3) to assess the group's knowledge about the problem or prior experiences that relate to the problem, (4) to select and utilize the appropriate content, and (5) to determine ways to evaluate the results of implemented plans.

The following is a sample discussion of a nursing care incident about which a patient-centered conference was conducted. It is not intended to be all-inclusive but is used to illustrate how a nurse-leader can conscientiously apply principles of teaching and learning (see Chapter 2) to bring about the desired goal of improving patient care through the use of patient-centered conferences. The participants in the sample conference are members of the nursing team in a newborn nursery setting. Each person participates in ways commensurate with his role and capability. General introductory activities and other material and comments not specifically illustrative have been deleted. What remains is the process and structure.

LVN: I am caring for Baby Lee in 317A. He was born at 2 A.M., was full term, and weighed 7 pounds. Everything was going along well until this morning when he began to breathe in a strange way. He became very restless, began to breathe with jerky respirations, and his ribs pulled in with every breath. Right after that he started to grunt, cough, and then turned blue. I was scared to death; I did what I could, and called for help. The team leader knew what to do, and he is breathing better now.

Leader: What do you believe are the problems in this situation?

LVN: Well, I'd surely like to know what went wrong with him and I'd like to know if I did the right thing.

Leader: Anything else?

Aide: What I want to know is what do we do if a baby goes bad like that when we are taking care of it!

All: (Indications of consensus.)

Leader: (To LVN) What have you decided is the problem for the group to consider now?

LVN: I think all of us should know what to do in case that happens again.

At this point the group has moved through the preliminary assessment period. The teaching and learning principle that *learner need and readiness influences content and rate of learning* was implemented by the leader. The group was taken through a process that identified their need and readiness to learn.

The nurse-leader then implemented the principles that *participation of the learner in setting learning goals makes learning activities meaningful and useful to the learner; and realistic behavioral goal setting enables selection of appropriate and meaningful content.* This was illustrated by the participation of the aide and LVN in stating and delineating the problem and in the group consensus about the topic for the conference. The established goal is realistic and behavioral and indicates to the nurse-leader the body of knowledge necessary to meet the goal. The teaching and learning principles about anxiety and motivation are implemented in this situation because the respiratory distress of Baby Lee has created the anxiety that members may not be able to meet a similar emergency situation.

PREDICTIVE PRINCIPLE: *Analyzing nursing care given in the light of established goals enables members to validate their behavior and to devise ways to improve nursing care.*

A member confronted with a problem while administering nursing care will react in some way. If the individual can describe his behavior in the nursing situation but is unable to give reasons for the care given, there is evidence of lack of understanding. Nursing care situations are ideal for assisting the members to increase in knowledge and understanding without jeopardizing their sense of personal worth.

There is no better way to implement the teaching and learning principle that *an obvious relationship between learning activities and stated goals increases the motivational value of the activity* than to discuss what was done by the person involved in the situation at the time of the incident.

In the case of Baby Lee the group was well aware of the overall goal areas for the care of all infants—observation, prevention, comfort, and nurturing. When the LVN observed signs and symptoms that deviated from normal, she acted in an attempt to restore the infant to the desired state of being. The immediate crisis for her was over, but unanswered questions remained, causing her to experience anxiety. Through verbal interaction the LVN shared with co-workers her behavior in the time of crisis.

Aide: (To LVN): What did you do when Baby Lee started having trouble?
LVN: First, I made sure there was nothing obstructing the air from getting into his lungs.
Aide: How did you do that?
LVN: I pressed my thumb down on his chin and opened his mouth to see if I could see any signs of obstruction. He had quite a bit of mucus but nothing more. Then I turned him on his side with his head brought forward to relax his throat as much as possible to allow the mucus to run out. By this time the team leader answered my call.
Leader: You did the right thing: An open airway is the first thing to look for.

The LVN's actions were a result of her previous knowledge and experience. She acted maturely, demonstrated an ability to function well under stress, and carried out nursing activities based on previously learned materials about the emergency care of the infant who had respiratory distress. The nurse-leader's comment on appropriate action implemented the teaching and learning principle that *rewards of recognition, praise, peer status, or valued gains are motivating and reinforcing factors facilitating learning rate, amount of retention, and degree of behavior change.* The recognition and praise validated and reinforced the appropriate action of the LVN and served as a vehicle for the members to devise ways to meet similar nursing emergencies and thus improve nursing care.

Validation served to help the LVN feel successful about handling the crisis, increased her confidence, lowered her anxiety, and readied the group to acquire additional information and move into the next stage of the learning process.

The LVN has completed the account of her experience. The leader's role now is that of teacher, because the LVN is unable to render the nursing care required in this situation.

Leader: When I arrived, I percussed the baby's posterior chest (illustrates the procedure with hands) before I suctioned him to loosen the secretions. He had quite a lot of thick material in him. This procedure will have to be done every 20 minutes or so.

Aide: Can we do that procedure?

Leader: No, the LVN and I will. Your part is to note if he appears to be in trouble again with his breathing; then call us right away. He is now in an Isolette with oxygen and an I.V.

LVN: Baby Lee is suspected of having hyaline membrane disease, which is a condition affecting the lungs. I know that it occurs mostly with premature babies. Baby Lee is full term. I would like to know more about the disease. Can we take it as our subject for the content conference?

Leader: All agreed? Fine. I will get some reading material together and make it available to you. Find out as much as you can before Thursday. In the meantime, I will tell you that Baby Lee's critical period is the next 48 hours. It is very important that he (1) be kept in the warmed Isolette with 40% oxygen, (2) be percussed and suctioned every 20 minutes, (3) have his umbilical catheter kept intact, (4) be watched carefully to see that his I.V. goes at 10 drops per minute, (5) have his respirations recorded and graphed every 15 minutes (more often if necessary), and (6) be observed for signs of change in color or severe distress.

The LVN and I will assume responsibility for the treatments. We want everyone to help us with observation. Each time you go by his Isolette, will you have a look at him with these things in mind? Should you have occasion to note these same symptoms that the LVN has described in an infant you are caring for, do just as she did. Make sure there is no obstruction, then turn the child on his side and bring his head forward and call for help.

The nurse-leader has given new information and set limits describing the patient's immediate needs and who is responsible for meeting those needs. This implements the teaching and learning principle that *structure, limits, and feedback provide an environment that promotes security and trust.*

The LVN now takes the lead by giving information she has acquired about the patient but is to her of less importance than was the immediate problem of Baby Lee's compromised respirations.

The group has requested an opportunity to learn more about hyaline membrane disease. The leader has applied the principle that *learning in real rather than contrived situations facilitates ease of learning and retention* and has been consistent in the philosophy of the value of learner participation in goal setting. The nurse-leader (1) made sure the group had enough information to function safely immediately, (2) set group expectations of nursing responsibilities for the next 48 hours to allay anxiety about the course of events before the more long-range goals could be met, and (3) established goals commensurate with group need for the next meeting.

Since the objective for the patient-centered conference was a behavioral goal, the evaluation of the conference is built into the objective itself. If group members demonstrate in their subsequent care of Baby Lee that they can function effectively within the limits and expectations discussed in the conference, learning will have occurred.

PREDICTIVE PRINCIPLE: *Formation of written nursing care plans from patient-centered conferences provides a central, continuous source of information.*

The nursing care plan is a written expression of the nursing process. A care plan is essential for the scheduling purposes and is generally made accessible to personnel through transcription. Where advisable, a copy of the care plans may be left with the client for his understanding, participation, fulfillment, and direction. Nursing care plans are best formulated from patient-centered, problem-oriented conferences. While it is conceivable that the leader could write a nursing care plan without consulting other persons, it is not recommended. The synthesis ensures a more comprehensive and accurate care plan. Furthermore, the care plan is more apt to be followed by client and care givers if they participate in its formation.

The patient-centered conference concerning Baby Lee is used as an example of transposing verbal communication into written form where vital content becomes accessible to all personnel involved with his care. Only those headings that have bearing on the case will be explored:

PHYSICIAN'S ORDERS

    Warmed Isolette with 40% oxygen
    Percuss and suction q. 20 min. or p.r.n.
    Heparin-saline sol. through umbilical catheter p.r.n.
    Sodium bicarbonate 3.75 Gm. or 44.6 mEq. in 50 ml. I.V., 10 gtts/min.
    Bennett respirator
    Record and graph resp. rate q. 15 min. q. ½ hr. or p.r.n.

PROTECTIVE MEASURES (NEEDS)

    Maintain controlled temperature of Isolette
    Keep open airway (observe for excessive mucus)
    Maintain prescribed flow of I.V. fluid
    Keep arterial catheter in place (may need to inject heparin quickly)
    Careful observation of color and breathing
    Keep on either side

PHYSICAL CARE (NURSING INTERVENTION)

    Position on either side with head in forward position
    Percuss and suction q. 20 min. or p.r.n.
    Observe closely for cyanosis (blueness), dyspnea (difficult breathing)

FAMILY

    Mother is highly anxious about child (is hospitalized postpartal in room 342)
    Mother may sit by Isolette as desired (physician's permission granted)
    Father anxious. Work phone, 282-5486; Home, 369-1182
    Grandmother, Mrs. Baxter (keeping three small children in their home)

It is quite likely than an infant in critical condition might require some religious ritual; in this event the notations would be made under the appropriate heading. Later, as the baby progressed, referrals might be made and other family needs identified that would be worked out through the care plan, such as parental teaching.

Nursing care plans, developed on a systematic basis, derived from careful analysis of patient needs, and structured in collaboration with all concerned individuals and groups enable clients and agencies efficiently and fully to utilize nursing manpower. The economics involved in planning and implementing patient care are just as important to the agency and patient as is the planning of personnel time and duties. Every coordinator of nursing services expends a considerable length of time planning time schedules for employees, patients, and families. The efficient use of the full abilities and potential of each employee with patient and family will result in maximum services for monies paid.

CONTENT CONFERENCES

Constant input of knowledge enables client and care givers more effectively to perform the tasks implicity and explicitly expected of them. One way of assuring participants opportunity to increase their learning is to provide them with time to meet for the sole purpose of exploring content. Traditionally, content conferences have been reserved for the novice, based on the premise that the student or nurse in a refresher program needs time set aside to concentrate on specific content.

When an aide, LVN, or nurse has completed the appropriate basic course, education has just begun. Self-development and incidental learning are growth producing. However, planned classes or content conferences furnish a vital and necessary link in the continuing education of nursing personnel.

The practice of nursing can be improved in an environment that encourages individuals and groups to investigate ways to prevent problems. The opportunity to improve care entices the member with an inquiring mind and a creative spirit to grow and to innovate better nursing practices. Nursing practiced in a setting where learning is treated as exciting as well as useful reaps the benefits of such an attitude through a continued upgrading of the quality of care given. Individuals who become interested in developing better nursing practices will not only improve in ability but also will, by example, generate interest in others to follow suit.

Content conferences, like patient-centered sessions, are usually held about once a week for a period of 30 minutes to one hour or at any convenient time where primary care is in practice. The scheduling and length of time varies with the type of nursing activity. However, adherence to the scheduled time indicates the importance of and commitment to the need for the conference. When pressures in the work situation occur or some member is not as well prepared as he would like to be, it may seem expedient to drop the meeting from the schedule with the intent of meeting at a "better time." Almost without exception, the more convenient time never arrives. Members who form the habit of keeping their commitments are usually productive.

The goal of a content conference is derived from any aspect of nursing that meets the need of the membership. The field is open to a broad range of subject matter. Medical concerns such as symptoms, pathology, laboratory results, clinical course of a disease, diagnostic test procedures, and pharmacologic data interest nursing personnel and influence nursing activities and judgments. Nursing content such as patient care or comfort problems, patient teaching needs, new technologic advancements, and preventive care are areas constantly in need of attention. Because of time allotment, all areas cannot be covered; if attempted, the conference would result in a general coverage of a number of problems with no appreciable gain in theoretical and practical understanding of what nursing involves. To ensure a successful content conference the subject matter must be (1) needed by the membership, (2) something that can be considered in the allotted time, and (3) adequately prepared prior to the meeting.

Leadership varies with each conference. Like the patient-centered conference, the initiator of the subject matter usually takes the lead. The amount of guidance and assistance needed to prepare for the conference will depend on the individual's capabilities. Often the leader will suggest sharing the responsibility for presentation of content. All group members are expected to contribute to the discussion. Content conferences need not restrict contributions to the members of the group involved; participation from any person—coordinator of nursing services, physician, social worker, or therapist, including the patient or family—may be included when feasible and appropriate.

PREDICTIVE PRINCIPLE: *Member participation in problem-solving processes during content conference results in desired knowledge being patterned into a meaningful whole.*

Participants come to content conferences having acquired a body of antecedent information. They are ready to fit their knowledge and understanding together to form predictive principles that can be used to prescribe nursing actions.

The need to learn more about hyaline membrane disease, expressed by the membership in the patient-centered conference on Baby Lee, will be continued as an example of the theory-building process in a content conference. The following is a model of a problem-solving process in a content conference:

LVN: (After giving a recall of background data about Baby Lee.) The definition of hyaline membrane disease is "a syndrome of neonatal distress, characterized by a hyaline-like material within the alveoli and bronchioles." This disease is very much like emphysema, in which bronchi in the lungs end in thin-walled air spaces (illustrates with chalk drawing).

The LVN has begun the conference by referring to content familiar to the group. Her next step is to introduce new information and then to make it meaningful by relating the facts to the more familiar condition (emphysema). Visual media assist the learning process. The LVN has applied the principle that *content that flows from the familiar to the unfamiliar provides a point of reference and promotes efficient grasping of material.*

Aide: Did you find out why the baby has this disease? I read that babies with hyaline membrane disease are usually premature, and Baby Lee is not.

LVN: Yes, I did. The specific cause of the disease is unknown, but it does occur frequently in two conditions. One is with premature babies, as we know, and the other occurs in babies born of mothers who have untreated diabetes mellitus.

Student: What about the mother? Has she been tested?

Leader: The doctor contacted her, and she had a blood test, which proved positive. Mrs. Lee was shocked to say the least, but is now learning all she can about the problem.

Members in this conference are concerning themselves with a real situation, which is never simple. Extraneous factors will enter in and must be considered if they are pertinent to the subject. These activities actualize the principle that *learning in real rather than contrived situations facilitates ease of learning and retention.*

LVN: Baby Lee's problems center around respirations. I have, with the help of the team leader, placed facts on the blackboard that will help us to see why Baby Lee is having problems. Will you help in deciding what they are? Anything you can add will be welcome.

Student: His carbon dioxide and oxygen combining powers indicate that acidosis is developing.

Aide: What does that mean?

Student: Interference with gas exchange in the lungs causes carbon dioxide retention.

The conference continues in an atmosphere of freedom, allowing facts and concepts to be exchanged and clarification of the learning structure to occur. The problem-solving process continues until the group has formulated principles pertinent to the situation and has developed nursing prescriptions supported by theory. The following is a sample of some of the formalizations as a result of group process.

PREDICTIVE PRINCIPLES	NURSING PRESCRIPTION
1. Poor heat regulation center prompts use of external control of temperature.	1. Warm Isolette.
2. Loosening tenacious pulmonary secretions facilitates breathing.	2. Percuss before suctioning to loosen pulmonary secretions.
3. Blood gas measurements indicate changing physiologic state.	3. Keep open arterial catheter (heparin-saline solution can be used).
4. The use of sodium bicarbonate I.V. combats acidosis.	4. Monitor closely.
5. In respiratory acidosis the use of positive pressure respirator promotes the blowing off of excessive CO_2.	5. Record and graph respiratory rate every half-hour or p.r.n.

PREDICTIVE PRINCIPLE: *Conferences held between nurse and client and/or significant others contribute to reciprocal development of care plans and lead to optimal health service for the client and satisfaction for the nurse.*

Assessment and maintenance provide the causal elements for primary care conferences. Patient-centered conferences are an effective means to bring together persons who can contribute to, or profit from analysis of the care plan. Conferences are usually initiated by the nurse but may originate from any one of the involved persons. The time, place, and length of the meeting is dependent on several circumstances—needs, urgency, and availability of resources, materials, and personnel. The purpose is to plan together problem-oriented client care. The nursing conference is equally applicable to singular needs and problems of the client as it is to complex situations requiring multiple consideration. The conference may be concerned with an initial assessment process or with an ongoing appraisal of a health situation. Members discuss the health of the client to arrive at a decision of what must be done to help resolve his problem and to delegate responsibility for the maintenance of health, evaluation and management of symptoms, and appropriate referrals.

To function logically and responsibly in an assessment conference the nurse must have knowledge and requisite skills in prescribing, providing care, and making referrals as appropriate.

The nurse-practitioner, sometimes labeled as the extended role or the primary nurse-practitioner, is a direct access nurse who has a one-to-one relationship with the client. Either the nurse or the client can initiate contact. Nursing responsibility includes history and physical examination, patient screening and referrals to appropriate physicians or other health workers, and nursing diagnosis and prescription, including counseling, care, and rehabilitation.

As health care is increasingly valued in our society, nurses are expected to take more responsibility for the delivery of health care, for coordinating preventive services, for initiating or participating in diagnostic screening, and for referring patients who require differential medical diagnoses and medical therapies.

The nurse-practitioner has moved into hospitals, assuming management of care for one or more selected patients mutually agreed upon by nursing and medical personnel and client. Responsibilities include screening patients and consultation and collaboration with client, peers, physicians, other health professionals, and appropriate community in planning and instituting health care programs. Most of these functions receive direction from and are benefited by conferences. With the added responsibilities placed on the nurse it is apparent that expertise in the conduct of conferences is important.

A report* submitted to the Secretary of Health, Education, and Welfare reviewing extended roles for nurses concluded that skills for the nurse-practitioner involve (1) eliciting and recording a health history, (2) making physical and psychosocial assessment, recognizing the range of "normal" and the manifestations of common abnormalities, (3) assessing the environment (family relationships, home, school, and work environments), (4) interpreting selected laboratory findings, (5) making diagnoses and choosing, initiating, and modifying selected therapies, (6) assessing community resources and needs for health care, (7) providing emergency treatment as appropriate, as in cardiac arrest, shock, or hemorrhage, and (8) providing appropriate information to the patient and his family about a diagnosis or plan of therapy.

Primary nursing care, a concept different from the above, involves one nurse's being responsible for the total nursing management of a patient or small group of patients. Nursing diagnosis and care plans based on a total and continuing assessment process are the vehicles for continuity and comprehensiveness. Primary nursing views the client as the center of action, focuses on him as a person, with the nurse having an increased opportunity for individual control and evaluation of functions.

---

*Nurs. Outlook 1:50-51, 1972.

In primary care, nurses assume considerably greater responsibility for delivery of health care services. Primary care nursing establishes a one-to-one nurse-patient relationship that can be experienced in any setting—home, community, or highly complex care context. The nurse assumes the role of client advocate. Primary nursing is a self-maintaining care system, open to the environment, with adaptive mechanisms for the single purpose of providing quality services. In this system, direct conferences are held between nurse and client and any other member who has significance to the client and his care.

In present practice, utilization of the primary nurse varies extensively. Community health nurses have always functioned with relative independence, but with physician collaboration, assessing problems of individuals and families, treating minor illnesses, referring patients for differential medical diagnosis, arranging for referrals to social service agencies and organizations, giving advice and counsel to promote health and prevent illness, supervising health regimens of normal pregnant women and of children, and working with health-related community action programs.

Team nursing, for the present, is one of the more common nursing care delivery systems and involves a group of people sharing responsibility for a number of patients. The team conference is the heart of this system. Nursing assessments, diagnosis, and care prescriptions are formulated by the group or team leader and furnish the guidelines for continuity and comprehensive practice. The team member assigned to a given client for a specified period of time is responsible for carrying out the plan and conferring with team members to revise the design.

PREDICTIVE PRINCIPLE: *Periodic care review conferences held with colleagues provide a mechanism for the nurse to validate care plans and maintain quality control.*

Each nurse, regardless of the system of nursing care delivery, is accountable for overall decisions about how the client is to receive attention. He is a decision maker in control of the quality of nursing care administered during his client contact. Additionally, primary nurses are responsible for the care giver in his absence. With the burgeoning knowledge in nursing, medicine, and related fields, to achieve comprehensiveness of health administration it is necessary to share knowledge and skills of a number of health experts, each of whom is prepared in a particular area. Together these individuals attempt adequately to meet the comprehensive needs of the client.

Review conferences between the nurse and such colleagues as other care givers, physician, nurse specialist, and supervisory nurse provide an excellent avenue for collegial validation and advisement, with an informal network of peer control and dialogue. During the conference each nurse presents the information on which the health plan is based and discusses the reasons for nursing prescriptions. Review conferences serve to increase the competency of the nurse, strengthen peer relationships, and maintain quality control necessary for the delivery of this health care system.

Nursing care conferences contribute to a sense of satisfaction in participants.

Relationships necessary for a professional level of responsibility and for the comprehensive care of the patient are developed. The dual concept of individual responsibility for the delivery of nursing services and care, with each nurse functioning at his own level of performance and each client participating in the implementation of his care plan to the extent of his motivation and level of competence, makes the practice of nursing challenging and exciting.

Utilization of the problem-solving process has taken a form that allows the learners to compile their facts and concepts into a meaningful pattern that is logical and sensible. Definite guidelines for evaluation of behaviors have been established.

REPORTING CONFERENCES

There is widespread agreement among nursing personnel on the importance of keeping the nurse-leader informed about ongoing activities. No leader can operate efficiently without sufficient knowledge about member activities. One of the most logical sources of information is the reporting conference, where events of the workday are shared by all those engaged in the administration of care. Members bring to the conference the work sheets upon which they have recorded the day's events. They verbally share pertinent information with the group. The coordinator of nursing services attends these sessions, for even though informed of major events throughout the shift, he usually has little opportunity to learn the many details discussed in the reporting conferences.

Reporting conferences have four major goals: (1) to report accurately and objectively relevant information, (2) to give reactions to situations when pertinent, (3) to evaluate the care in the light of objectives, and (4) to update the nursing care plans to ensure continuity of care for the client and family.

Listening is the primary task of the nurse-leader in reporting sessions. He must be a critical listener and be able to make judgments about the material being presented. The tools used to aid in this task are the leader's work sheet, a record of the physician's orders, awareness of client's reactions, nursing prescriptions, and knowledge, understanding, and intuition. As with the instructional conference, each member is encouraged to listen and record appropriate data about all patients or families for whom they are responsible.

The leader will utilize the information received in the reporting conference in finalizing action for the day, in recording data in patients' records, in giving the change-of-shift report to the oncoming staff, and in making plans for the next day.

Many predictive principles that have been proposed for all conferences have direct application to report giving. Prior preparation by all members, attention to behavioral messages, and paced and systematic presentation are of equal importance in the summarizing period.

PREDICTIVE PRINCIPLE: *Directions given to conferees before report reveal expectations the leader has for the members.*

Because situations vary in nursing, it is difficult to establish a set of criteria for reporting information. In primary care, for example, expectations for client(s) and nurse will be mutually agreed upon, with guidance from the leader. In acute situations the member must report many details; while in health care centers where the occupants' stay is long-term, or in the home, much routine information can be omitted. It is the leader's task to inform the members of the amount and kind of information desired. For example, a nurse-leader might begin by saying, "When I call on you, will you tell us please how the patient ate, his degree of ambulation, how he tolerated his treatments, and anything you believe to be important for us to know?"

This procedure sounds simple, but complications may occur. The average staff member usually gives routine information but may not be clear on what additional data to report. In many cases the worker's past nursing experience and educational background limit the extent of his reporting. Just prior to the conference, for example, an aide may have noted casually one of the patients assigned to him looked a little pale while ambulating in the hall. The worker did not consider this to be significant enough to report. The next day, when the patient was discovered slumped on the floor, the observation became significant to the aide and was reported.

There will be occasions when incidents that have proved troublesome to the member will be deleted from the report. The worker may not want to risk criticism, especially if he feels the incident or problem is a result of his mistake or poor judgment.

If something has been omitted from a report, the ultimate accountability lies with the leader. It is his task to prepare the members for their roles and to maintain an atmosphere where free exchange of information can occur. Preoccupation with fixing blame consumes time and energy better spent on solving the problems.

Continuing training, practice, and review, as necessary, will help nurses and clients mature in ability to select appropriate information and to report clearly and accurately.

Reports lend themselves to the use of tape recorders. Clarification and elucidation can be made after listening to the tape and before the reporting nurse departs.

GENERAL PROBLEMS CONFERENCES

One of the more difficult roles for the nurse-leader in conference sessions is to cope with feelings, both his own and those expressed by members. Control of one's feelings is held in personal, social, and cultural esteem by North American society. The individual is expected to maintain "proper" control of his feelings and also must act in a way that enables others to maintain theirs. Participants usually strive to convey precisely the feeling they believe others expect of them at a given time and place. Preoccupation with this goal may result in the neglect of the prescribed focus of attention.

Any work assignment has problems and emergencies. The way these problems are handled determines the amount and kind of feelings that will be built up in an individual. Many days are filled with one situation after another that build up tension in the person until he "travels on his nerves."

Members in conference sessions do not always operate as a "happy family." Because of individual interests, clashes occur between client, the health giving membership, and management. The nurse is not expected to be a psychiatrist, only to develop the ability to sense feelings and to understand and apply principles of effective interpersonal relationships when they are needed.

PREDICTIVE PRINCIPLE: *Sharing of feelings through conferences unifies and integrates the membership and allows work to progress.*

In work groups, members sometimes have little in common except that they are drawn together by joint enterprise. The task of becoming spontaneously involved in conference activity when it is a job expectation places the individual in a delicate position. Expressions of like feelings as well as those of alienation will be easier for some than for others.

These meetings are directly related to the administration of patient care. They should be scheduled often enough to keep the members in tune with one another. Interpersonal maintenance for goal accomplishment is a legitimate enterprise. A meeting should be called by the leader or any member anytime problems arise that hinder the communication process and therefore reduce work efficiency and effectiveness.

Reasons for tense situations may range from prejudice of one member against another to lack of consideration for the total membership by one individual. For example, problems may be created when a member announces openly that he plans to use all his accrued sick time because he is "never sick." His frequent absences without notice cause gaps in patient care and overloads for the remaining members, and hostility and anger result.

An alternative action for the above situations is open expressions of feelings about the behavior and its consequences in a feelings conference. In this way, feelings are expressed openly and handled. Until these feelings are relieved, there will be barriers to communications. Positive relationships need recognition and reinforcement on a continuous basis. It becomes easy to slip into the habit of dealing with crisis situations and to fail to acknowledge those behaviors that keep nursing practice on an even keel.

Expression of feelings becomes easier in the sharing process when one knows what the other is doing and feeling. The "feeling of knowing" is an emotional by-product of communication and makes the difference between the person who feels secure and the one who is anxious.

Development of a climate conducive to fostering collaborative interdependent and independent activity requires time, involvement, and concerted effort by each member. The operation of effective nursing process depends upon the maintenance of open, trusting relationships among the participants. If problems are acknowledged and faced frankly, the chances for a remedy are far greater than if ignored and allowed to fester.

PREDICTIVE PRINCIPLE: *Understanding and management of group behavior require ability to predict the processes through which feelings and meanings are transmitted among group members.*

Investigators of small-group process have found group members address more communication to individuals whose opinions are extreme than to the more conforming members. For instance, an individual group member might believe that the care givers have an obligation to urge hospital management to serve patients their meals upon request. If the majority opinion differs greatly from that of the dissentor, the group will exert pressure on the member in an effort to get him to change his opinion. Evidence shows that communication of feelings back to the instigator will reduce the intensity of feelings.

These findings make it possible for the members to pick up cues in behavior when they occur and to recognize the process as it unfolds. Another illustration will prove helpful. Probably the most common feeling expressed in conferences is that of pressure. Nurses seem to be particularly susceptible to pressure because the tasks are numerous, varied, and very often complex. The leader is frequently confronted with a member who is frustrated and angry and who vents his feelings in negative terms. "I have to be everywhere at once, and everything to everybody!" "There are not enough hours in the day; I have to do everything around here." "I'm still not caught up; I don't have time to sit in here and talk!" These feelings can be decreased if activities are put on a priority basis and the group shares the responsibility for the necessary ongoing work. Clear identification of anger and attempts to resolve the causes openly can effectively reduce member hostility and give the leader the opportunity to explore feelings with the individual concerned. If the discussion reveals duplication of effort, lack of organization, or, in fact, too large an assignment, adjustments can be made in the structure or perhaps even in the system of care. Failure to change the feelings may result in their intensification and transmission to other members.

The real significance of the "contagion" theory of feelings is that members recognize the impact they have on one another. Feelings of acceptance, caring, trust, and security will be transmitted when they exist, just as feelings of rejection, anger, hate, or hostility will be communicated in spite of attempts to hide them from the group. It is important to establish the rule among conferees that when feelings are interfering with the work of the group, they must dealt with.

PREDICTIVE PRINCIPLE: *Involvement in group process results in specific gains or losses for the individual member.*

Rewards may take the form of such intangibles as prestige, recognition, or affection. The conditions or rules that govern the awarding of the payoff will have important motivational consequences for the members and for the functioning of the group as a whole.

Each person wants to feel that his individual contribution to cooperative endeavor is significant and identifiable. Group work, however, can subjugate some members to others unnecessarily unless steps are taken to offset this possibility.

In group process, "role blurring" is encouraged, in which emphasis is placed on outcomes of the group rather than on the status of the individual. The leader works with health care personnel to provide opportunity for each individual to expand his physical and mental energies to his fullest potential. In the process, personal achievements are recognized and the worth of the person is reinforced, but individual recognition does not take priority over group accomplishment.

If position or salary increments depend on such individual performances as the number of beds made or procedures accomplished, group effort is apt to diminish. If, on the other hand, a group is operating under a policy whereby each person's benefits depend directly on the group's performance, the members will want to engage in whatever behaviors they believe will contribute to this end (working hard, helping others, and making suggestions about ways to improve the group's efficiency).

In industry a reward system of this kind operates most frequently in plant operations where salable items are the end result of effort and dividends include monetary gain. In nursing, patients are the end product; when they have benefited from the coordinated efforts of a group, tangible reward to all members, beyond established policy, are not forthcoming. The care giver's motivation, then, centers around achievement of satisfaction in a job well done, acknowledgment by management, and patients' appreciation.

Involvement in group activity does not negate the autonomy and individual accountability reflected in the role of the primary care nurse. This leader has the freedom to move in and out of groups as necessary to the needs of the client and dynamics of the nursing care plan.

APPLICATION OF PREDICTIVE PRINCIPLES IN COMMUNICATIONS

RN, Mrs. Turner, recently joined a nursing group on the rehabilitative unit. Her former experience included ten years working with paraplegic patients in another part of the country. She is convinced her knowledge and experience far surpasses that of any other members. The RN completes her assignments by herself, communicating as little as possible with the members, who have countered with expressions of hostility.

PROBLEM	PREDICTIVE PRINCIPLES	PRESCRIPTIONS
Noncommunicative member	In retrospect: Preassessment of individual and group knowledges, skills, and expectations establishes base-line data for measurement of progress or change.	
	The nature of leadership practices determines the type of group process that will evolve	Leader will have conference with RN; state observed behavior and problems that have arisen because of aloofness from others. Assist RN to recognize the influence one member's
	Understanding and management of group behavior require ability to predict the processes through which feelings and meanings are transmitted among group members.	

PROBLEM	PREDICTIVE PRINCIPLES	PRESCRIPTIONS
Noncommunicative member—cont'd	The extent of involvement of each group member determines the proficiency of the group.	action has on the entire group and the responsibility of group to discuss the problem.
	Circumstance and member capability determine the type of direction to be communicated.	Arrange meeting with all members; conduct so meeting will be a discussion of cause for behavior; encourage open communication (not a punitive session).
	Positive interdependent relationships facilitate group cohesiveness and achievement of goals with speed and efficiency.	
	Perceiving negative feedback enables group members to become aware of others' responses to them and their effects on the group and to evaluate goal attainment and to modify behavior accordingly.	Make positive plans with member for reinforcing positive behavior.

BIBLIOGRAPHY
BOOKS

Amidon, E. J., and Hough, J. B., editors: Interaction analysis: theory, research and application, Reading, Mass., 1967, Addison-Wesley Publishing Co., Inc.

Banathy, B. H.: Instructional systems, Palo Alto, Calif., 1968, Fearon Publishers.

Bell, G. D.: Organizations and human behavior, Englewood Cliffs, N. J., 1967, Prentice-Hall, Inc.

Bloom, B. S., editor: Taxonomy of educational objectives: the classification of educational goals. Handbook I. Cognitive domain, New York, 1956, David McKay Co., Inc.

Bloom, B. S., et al.: Handbook on formative and summative evaluation of student learning, New York, 1971, McGraw-Hill Book Co.

Bower, F. L.: The process of planning nursing care: a theoretical model, St. Louis, 1972, The C. V. Mosby Co.

Carkhuff, R. R., and Berenson, B. G.: Beyond counseling and therapy, New York, 1967, Holt, Rinehart and Winston, Inc.

Carlson, E.: Learning through games: a new approach to problem solving, Washington, D.C., 1969, Public Affairs Press.

Cartwright, D., and Zander, A., editors: Group dynamics—research and theory, ed. 3, New York, 1968, Harper & Row, Publishers.

Combs, A., et al.: Helping relationships: basic concepts for the helping professions, Boston, 1972, Allyn & Bacon, Inc.

Fast, J.: Body language, New York, 1970, J. B. Lippincott Co.

Gage, N. L., editor: Handbook of research on teaching. A project of the American research association, Chicago, 1963, Rand McNally & Co.

Gagne, R. W.: The condition of learning, New York, 1965, Holt, Rinehart and Winston, Inc.

Glasser, W.: Schools without failure, New York, 1969, Harper & Row, Publishers.

Glasser, W.: Reality therapy: a new approach to psychiatry, New York, 1965, Harper & Row, Publishers.

Goffman, E.: Interaction ritual: essays on face-to-face behavior, New York, 1967, Anchor Press.

Gordon, A. K.: Games for growth: educational games in the classroom, Palo Alto, Calif., 1970, Science Research Associates, Inc.

Gulley, H. E.: Discussion, conference, and group process, ed. 2, New York, 1968, Holt, Rinehart and Winston, Inc.

Harris, T. A.: I'm OK—You're OK, New York, 1973, Harper & Row, Publishers.

Inbar, M., editor: Simulation and games: an international journal of theory, design and research, Beverly Hills, Calif., 1970, Sage Publications, Inc.

Krathwohl, D. R., et al.: Taxonomy of educational objectives: the classification of educational goals. Handbook II. Affective domain, New York, 1964, David McKay Co., Inc.

Litterer, J. A.: Organizations: systems, control

and adaptation, ed. 2, New York, 1969, John Wiley & Sons, Inc., vol. 2.

Little, D., and Carnevali, D.: Nursing care planning, 1969, J. B. Lippincott Co.

Luft, J.: Group processes, an introduction to group dynamics, Palo Alto, Calif., 1970, National Press Books.

Mager, R. F.: Developing attitude toward learning, Belmont, Calif., 1968, Fearon Publishers.

Mager, R. F.: Preparing instructional objectives, Palo Alto, Calif., 1962, Fearon Publishers.

Marram, G. D.: The group approach in nursing practice, St. Louis, 1973, The C. V. Mosby Co.

McAshan, H. H.: Writing behavioral objectives: a new approach, New York, 1970, Harper & Row, Publishers.

McGrath, J. E., and Irwin, A.: Small group research, New York, 1966, Holt, Rinehart and Winston, Inc.

Pohl, M. L.: The teaching function of the nursing practitioner, ed. 2, Dubuque, Iowa, 1973, William C. Brown Co., Publishers.

Ruesch, J.: The observer and the observed: human communication theory. In Grinker, R. R., editor: Toward a unified theory of human behavior, New York, 1956, Basic Books, Inc., Publishers.

Ruesch, J.: General theory of communication. In Arieti, S., editor: American handbook of psychiatry, New York, 1961, W. W. Norton & Co., Inc.

Ruesch, J., and Bateson, G.: Communication: the social matrix of psychiatry, New York, 1968, W. W. Norton & Co., Inc.

Ruesch, J., Shannon, A., and Weaver, W.: The mathematical theory of communication, Urbana, Ill., 1949, University of Illinois Press.

Simon, A., editor: Classroom interaction newsletter, Philadelphia, 1970, Research for Better Schools.

Tansey, P. J., and Unwin, D.: Simulation and gaming in education, London, 1969, Methuen Educational Ltd.

Twelker, P. A., editor: Instructional simulation systems: an annotated bibliography, Corvallis, Oregon, 1969, Oregon State University Press.

PERIODICALS

Chopra, A.: Motivation in task oriented groups, J. Nurs. Admin., pp. 55-60, Jan.-Feb., 1973.

Combs, A. W., et al.: Florida studies in the helping professions, University of Florida Social Science Monograph, No. 37, 1969.

Dickoff, P. J., and Wiedenbach, J.: Theory in a practice discipline. Part I. Practice oriented theory, Nurs. Res. 17(5):415-35, 1968.

Gallagher, J. J., and Aschner, M. J.: A preliminary report on an analysis of classroom interaction, The Merrill Palmer Quarterly of Behavior and Development, 9:3, 1963.

Jehring, J. J.: Motivational problems in the modern hospital, J. Nurs. Admin., pp. 35-47, Nov.-Dec., 1972.

Lewis, G. K.: Communication, a factor in meeting emotional crisis, Nurs. Outlook 13:36-39, 1965.

Little, D., and Carnevali, D.: The nursing care planning system, Nurs. Outlook 19:164-167, 1971.

Palmer, M. E.: Patient care conference: an opportunity for meeting staff needs, J. Nurs. Admin., pp. 47-53, Mar.-Apr., 1973.

Smith, D.: Writing objectives as a nursing practice skill, Am. J. Nurs. 71(2):319-320, 1971.

Stevens, L. F.: Nurse-patient discussion groups, Am. J. Nurs. 63(12):67-69, 1963.

Teaching patients and use of the self in clinical practice, Nurs. Clin. North Am. 6:4, Dec., 1971.

Vaill, P. B.: Management language and management action, Calif. Management Rev., pp. 51-58, Oct., 1967.

Veninga, R.: Communications: a patient's eye view, Am. J. Nurs. 73(2):320-322, 1973.

Zander, A., et al.: Unity of group, identification with group and self-esteem of members, J. Pers. 28:463-465, 1960.

CHAPTER FOUR

Predictive principles for delegating authority

AGENCY STRUCTURE

A working knowledge of the organizational structure of the health agency in which the nurse-leader works promotes appropriate delegation of responsibility, for organizational structure determines the amount and degree of authority that can be delegated.

Delegation of authority to the agency level closest to the job to be done leads to overall organizational effectiveness and decision making.

Understanding the categories and roles of nursing personnel enables the delegator to select the type and number of personnel appropriate for the job.

JOB DESCRIPTIONS, POLICIES, AND PROCEDURES

Written descriptions of policies, procedures, and/or guidelines by which an employee may handle situations when they occur promote ease of operation for the care giver and control of the authority delegated by the nurse-leader.

Member participation in the formulation of policies, job descriptions, and procedures increases member cooperation.

The philosophy and policies of a health agency determine the pattern of nursing care delivery system to be provided.

Guidelines such as established channels, methods, and provision for communication within an agency enable the nurse-leader to delegate tasks and authority appropriately.

Clear lines of communication promote morale among organization members and enhance goal accomplishment.

Reactions to stress influence efficiency of performance in the work situation.

INVESTMENT OF AUTHORITY

The nurse-leader's belief that ultimate accountability lies with him determines the scope and limitations he sets for his leadership.

ASSIGNMENT MAKING

A thorough problem-oriented approach to patient-centered care enables the care giver to develop effective nursing care plans for the client or patient.

Assignment of authority necessitates a willingness on the part of the nurse-leader to relinquish authority.

A sufficient number of prepared personnel allows effective delegation of authority to meet organizational and patient needs.

Matching the abilities of care givers to the jobs to be done increases work productivity and individual job satisfaction.

Centralization of information storage and information giving and retrieval systems allows for efficient assessment, delegation, and implementation of tasks.

Clear and concise directions enhance task delegation.

A balance between variety and consistency of assignment increases worker's motivation and productivity.

Consideration for each care giver's preferences and areas of expertise influences morale.

A systematic planning process predisposes effective delegation.

Assignments that have clearly defined standards and goals provide a basis for measurement of outcome.
Frequent comparison of actual performance with criteria determines the quality of care and the level of actual performance.

One of the most important facets of a nurse-leader's job is that of delegating authority. Productivity can be maximized through wise delegation of responsibility to appropriate persons. These individuals may be patients, family members, or other nursing care givers. Delegation carries with it the responsibility for appropriately guiding and supervising the efforts of others toward the attainment of specific goals. Traditionally nurses have assumed every conceivable task in the hospital or health agency. In addition to nursing they have repaired equipment, made supplies, and served as housekeepers, clerks, and secretaries. It is neither realistic nor desirable to assume that a nurse is prepared to, or should, function well in all capacities. From an administrative point of view, diversion of the professional nurse's skills to tasks other than nursing is a costly and inefficient use of a professional person's time.

The major responsibility of a nurse-leader is to provide care to a patient (or client), or to a group of patients, or to serve with ancillary workers and other significant care givers in the role of validator, catalyst, decision maker, and controller of nursing care quality. The ability to perform these roles assumes that every care giver collaborates and carries his share of responsibility. Inherent in the philosophy of delegating responsibility is a commitment to the proposition that each nursing care giver must be entrusted with some degree of responsibility for the tasks under his jurisdiction and that he has the authority to act, thus making him accountable for his nursing actions. This assumes that the nurse-leader must possess knowledge and skills commensurate with the responsibility of organizing and directing activities and making nursing care decisions that affect others.

An effective leader is an organizer. Wise delegation of authority can result in an organization that is effective in accomplishing objectives with conservation of time and materials and can produce the greatest return in job satisfaction. The optimal performance of any assignment depends to a large extent upon the formulation of definite plans based on the organization's objectives. Nurse-leaders have become increasingly aware of the need for guidance in selecting the methods of delegation and of the need for specific tools to prepare them for the task of guiding themselves and others. Research in human motivation, leadership, communication, and employee development has contributed substantially to the understanding of this function.

AGENCY STRUCTURE

What the employer expects from an employee is based on the policies or objectives that guide the enterprise as determined by the philosophy and standards set by the organization. Most health institutions possess a common basis for existence: to serve the health needs of the public. This goal is reached in accordance with the type of health requirements of the agency's clients. Inherent in meeting health needs are (1) administering patient care, (2) educating health agency personnel and the public, (3) engaging in research, and (4) protecting the health of the public. The type of agency determines its major emphasis. Each type of agency structure shapes or sets limits to the type of operative goals likely to prevail, although there will be much variation within each type.

PREDICTIVE PRINCIPLE: *A working knowledge of the organizational structure of the health agency in which the nurse-leader works promotes appropriate delegation of responsibility, for organizational structure determines the amount and degree of authority that can be delegated.*

There are basically three organizational structures in health agencies—official, voluntary, and proprietary. Each focuses its attention on its own special clientele. *Official agencies* operate under federal, state, county, or city direction to provide health benefits for the large segment of the population covered in some way by legislation. This group is made up of psychiatric patients, war veterans, members of the armed services and their families, the disabled, and, most recently, senior citizens. Tax moneys provide the primary source of income.

Voluntary agencies are nonprofit corporations that serve the public according to the recipient's financial situation and/or according to the availability of services to the public through other means. Basic support for voluntary agencies depends upon monetary gifts for an important part of their capital and operating budget. Officially, trustees are the ultimate authority in voluntary hospitals. They do not necessarily exercise their legal powers, but when they do, there is no question about their authority. Since board members are drawn from distinctive social groups in the community, they may be oriented toward service for a religious, ethnic, economic, or age group. Such orientations have operative goals that affect standards and techniques of care, priority or services, access to care, relations with other organizations, and directions and rate of development.

Proprietary agencies are privately owned corporations operated for profit by independent owners. Proprietary health agencies function under the direction of individuals or groups of individuals, such as a corporation or a board of trustees; however, the formal authority structure may flow back and forth between central domination (individual owners or boards of trustees) to control by providers of care, depending on changes in goals and authority figures. Accordingly, agencies will vary with regard to personnel practices, client services, growth, and emphasis upon quality or quantity of care. Many proprietary agencies receive supplementary funds through private and public funding for provision of health care, research, and special services and are in a position to provide financial assistance to eligible clients. The transplanting of human organs is an example of a service that is financially out of reach for the average citizen but can be made available by special arrangement.

With the advent of the independent nurse practitioner all costs for nursing services are not generated from the agency in which the service is rendered. Reimbursement for special nursing services is arranged by contract between the nurse and the client or between representing agents, a system similar to that used by visiting nurse associations.

Agency organization

Whenever an enterprise expands beyond the size that can be effectively managed by one person, a grouping of activities is necessary, and departmentalization occurs. Typical organizational structure of a health agency includes a governing board, a director of the agency, and directors of business affairs, supportive services, and medical and nursing services. As expansion of the facility takes place, organizational structure grows both vertically and horizontally.

Nursing services are set up according to the guidelines established by the agency. The basis for departmentalization usually falls into three categories: territory, function, and service. *Departmentalization by territory* is advocated where nursing measures can be carried out with economy and expediency of operation. Establishment of clinics for migratory workers within their camps is one example; rehabilitative services for geriatric patients in hospitals or clinics is another. *Departmentalization by function* is usually based on the service to be rendered and the type of equipment involved. Activities are grouped according to the task being done. The need for heavy specialized equipment or a need for serial use of different equipment makes departmentalization by function desirable. Operating rooms, blood banks, cardiac catheterization, inhalation therapy, or central supply departments are in this category. *Departmentalization according to medical diagnosis or type of nursing service needed* is the most widely accepted practice in health agencies. It is a basis for structuring a complex organization that includes a variety of job activities. Medical, surgical, pediatric, and obstetric areas illustrate departmentalization by medical diagnosis. Intensive care, ambulatory care, convalescent care, and outpatient services illustrate departmentalization by type of nursing service required. There is some overlap in the three types of departmentalization, and the priority needs usually determine the category assignment.

PREDICTIVE PRINCIPLE: *Delegation of authority to the agency level closest to the job to be done leads to overall organizational effectiveness and decision making.*

Delegation of authority can be centralized or decentralized. A *centralized* organization is one in which detailed and comprehensive planning is done by the chief executive or by a group of high-level managers. Under this structure all nursing assignments are issued from the central nursing office. Centralized organizations tend to deemphasize the human element in favor of accomplishment of purpose and to encourage close supervision of personnel at every level.

A *decentralized organization* is one in which operating decisions are made by the people closest to the situation. As health agencies move from small, centrally controlled operations to large, complex corporations, the need for decentralization of control increases. The intent of decentralized nursing service is to bring decision-making authority, responsibility, and accountability to an operational level. A nurse-leader's major responsibility is to have the client's nursing needs met in a cost effective manner. This is accomplished by reducing the degree of vertical control held at the top level and by developing increased horizontal communications at lower levels. A health agency that operates under the philosophy of decentralized power expects the director of nurses to delegate authority to supervisors. The supervisors will place responsibility in the hands of head nurses, and the head nurses will give staff nurses the opportunity to plan, direct, and guide the operation of nursing care.

Occupations in which individuals traditionally work independently usually carry with them managerial responsibilities. The work done by pathologists, radiologists, directors of medical or nursing services, or supervisors, for example, necessitates hours of individual activity but may also involve a variety of associations with personnel. On the other hand, some situations may dictate a narrow span of management, such as the nurse-leader directing the work of a small group of personnel comprising a nursing team. In all cases the employee's preparation and experience and the type of service to be rendered influence the amount and degree of authority that can be delegated.

PREDICTIVE PRINCIPLE: *Understanding the categories and roles of nursing personnel enables the delegator to select the type and number of personnel appropriate for the job.*

Categories of nursing personnel are many and vary with each employing agency. It is impossible to delineate clearly among services rendered by each group because of differences in standards and requirements on the national, state, and local levels. In general, nursing personnel is comprised of those who have had both formal and informal preparation.

Nurses' aides are usually trained on the job to perform unskilled services in private homes or health agencies under the supervision of a registered nurse or a physician. Formal preparation usually consists of a few weeks of training in which the aides spend several hours a day learning from classroom demonstration, followed by supervised experience caring for patients in the employing agency. The extent of the training period is dependent on the philosophy and in-service educational program of the agency. Most nurses' aides administer hygienic care and perform such procedures as taking vital signs and tabulating oral intake and output. As health agencies become aware that nurses' aides are not cost effective, fewer and fewer nurses in this category are being employed.

Licensed Practical Nurses (LPN) or *Licensed Vocational Nurses (LVN)* may or may not have had formal training in a school designed for that purpose. LPNs or LVNs who are licensed by the state to practice fall into two categories. First, there are those who have received licensure by waiver upon proof of a specific number of years of satisfactory nursing practice and have taken a definite number of class hours as prescribed by the licensing board. Vocational or practical nurses who have received licensure by waiver are most often those who have been working as nurses' aides for years and have taken advantage of the opportunity to advance to the next step.

The second group of LPNs or LVNs are those who are licensed to practice in their state upon completion of a prescribed course of study in an approved vocational school. These courses are offered either through an adult education board or under the auspices of a junior or community college. The LPN or LVN program varies in length and prepares the graduate to function in the home or health agency under the supervision of a physician or registered nurse. The LVN or LPN who falls in this second group provides nursing care to patients with simple nursing problems but in more complex situations than does the licensed practical nurse who has not had benefit of formal training in planning, implementing, and evaluating nursing care.

According to the statement of functions for the licensed practical nurse adopted by the Board of Directors for the American Nurses' Association in January, 1970, the LPN promotes effectiveness of the employing health agency through contacts with patients' relatives, fosters cooperative effort with all personnel involved in patient care, and utilizes community resources and relationships to enable the public to have a better understanding of health services.

Registered nurses are those who are licensed by their state to practice nursing skills in hospitals, military services, offices, clinics, private practice, homes, and in the community under the supervision of a licensed physician. Minimal requirements for the RN are that preparation be in a school with an associate of arts or baccalaureate degree program in nursing accredited by the state. According to the Curriculum Content Committee of the Associate Degree Seminar of the Western Council on Higher Education for Nursing in 1967, the *associate of arts degree* graduates render quality nursing care. They are not prepared to assume administrative responsibilities. The graduate is able to function with some degree of independence as a giver of primary nursing care. In some places, collaboration with or the supervision of an experienced professional nurse is required. Associate degree graduates are prepared to assume responsibility for their own growth within the profession of nursing.

The beginning practitioner (1) carries out nursing functions directly related to patient care, including participation in implementing the physician's therapeutic plan (for example, by administering medications and treatments), (2) renders direct patient care in nursing situations requiring nursing judgment and recognizes those situations that require a higher degree of nursing expertise, (3) gives patient care that demonstrates knowledge of the nursing principles taught in all courses in the associate degree nursing program, (4) functions as a member of the nursing care team and as such may direct and guide other team members who have less education and experience, and (5) recognizes the client's need for instruction related to health and takes action to provide the instruction.

Diploma program graduates are prepared (1) to function as a generalist in hospitals and similar community institutions and (2) to provide nursing care to patients and to engage in therapeutic, rehabilitative, and preventive activities on behalf of individual patients and groups of patients.*

The graduate of a *baccalaureate degree* program (B.S., R.N.) (1) engages

---

*Adapted from a program developed by an ad hoc committee and accepted by the National League for Nursing Council of Diploma Programs, May, 1971.

in direct patient care and is a skilled observer and participant, (2) functions as a teacher and as a responsible informant of health practices, (3) functions as a leader-supervisor of members of health groups, (4) functions as a collaborator and as an effective member of the immediate health team, serves as interpreter of nursing activities to allied professionals in planning optimal health programs, aids other members of the health group in carrying out research, and serves as interpreter of nursing activities to groups outside the professional health groups, and (5) functions as an inquiring person.*

The nurse's role has expanded to include the *nurse practitioner*. A definition supported by the American Nurses' Association in 1971† defines the nurse practitioner as one who has completed a program of study leading to competence as a registered nurse in an expanded role and whose responsibility encompasses (1) obtaining a health history, (2) assessing health-illness status, (3) entering a person into the health care system, (4) sustaining and supporting persons who are impaired, infirm, and ill during programs of diagnosis and therapy, (5) managing a medical care regimen for acute and chronically ill patients within established standing orders, (6) aiding in restoring persons to wellness and maximum function, (7) teaching and counseling persons about health and illness, (8) supervising and managing care regimens of normal pregnant women, (9) helping parents in guidance of children with a view to their optimal physical and emotional development, (10) counseling and supporting persons with regard to the aging process, (11) aiding people and their survivors during the dying process, and (12) supervising assistants to nurses. To date, no consensus has been reached as to the appropriate responsibilities of a nurse practitioner.

Differentiation of roles is in process. Each of the educational programs emphasizes technical competence and skill. Each adds the dimensions of problem solving and judgment. The thread of responsibility is inherent in all statements. But one major weakness is the lack of clarity in delineation of roles in the area of leadership. The reality of the nursing situation is that graduates of all LPN or LVN and RN programs are expected to function as nurse-leaders in some capacity. Graduates of programs that do not provide theory and practice in leadership find themselves in a difficult situation, for they are expected to assume jobs for which they are unprepared.

Students of nursing often meet practicum requirements by becoming members of nursing staffs. The philosophy and objectives of the nursing school must be in harmony with the health agency providing the student an opportunity to practice. Preplanning sessions take place between the instructor and those who will be working with the students to ensure smooth matriculation from school to health agency. Student schedules, such as assignment to a ward for a prescribed number of hours over a period of weeks on certain days, create challenges for the nurse-leader making such assignments. The nurse-leader learns

---

*Adapted from a program developed by a special interest committee of the Baccalaureate Degree Seminar of the Western Council on Higher Education for Nursing, April, 1968.
†From Marion Murphy, Ph.D., Chairman, Commission on Nursing Education, the American Nurse Association.

what assignment the instructor desires for the students and reconciles the needs of the students with the responsibilities of the unit for nursing care of patients.

JOB DESCRIPTIONS, POLICIES, AND PROCEDURES

Clearly defining the exact nature and the limits of authority for each member in an agency not only provides structure for modes of operation but also promotes role identification by workers, sets boundaries, and avoids the possibility of task duplication.

PREDICTIVE PRINCIPLE: *Written descriptions of policies, procedures, and/or guidelines by which an employee may handle situations when they occur promote ease of operation for the care giver and control of the authority delegated by the nurse-leader.*

PREDICTIVE PRINCIPLE: *Member participation in the formulation of policies, job descriptions, and procedures increases member cooperation.*

A sense of personal involvement is created when an individual is given the responsibility for participating in formulation of policies that concern him. Personal involvement results in a feeling of belonging and a sense of importance in the employee. Participation in the establishment of policies helps the member feel his contributions are of value. It is not feasible for a health agency to invite each employee to assist with the formulation of all controlling issues, but through the various mechanisms, personnel representing all levels can have a part in most decisions. Each department within an agency can send elected members to policy and procedure meetings to represent the thinking of the group. Members who have had a part in determining both the qualifications required for a job and the procedure for implementing that job are better able to use their capabilities productively and with assurance.

The task of delegating responsibility is lightened for the nurse-leader when affected others have had a part in investing the leader with the right to guide them in the performance of their work. Job descriptions, policies, and procedures become dynamic for working groups when the content is reviewed on a regular basis and changes are made in accordance with increased knowledge and understanding. Investigating current practices and research in comparable settings and studying policies and procedures recommended by licensing associations for professional groups enable the establishment of guidelines to be an ongoing process, that is, one in which guidelines are constantly being revised to reflect current nursing care needs.

PREDICTIVE PRINCIPLE: *The philosophy and policies of a health agency determine the pattern of nursing care delivery system to be provided.*

There are many ways to deliver nursing care. No one mode of delivery is better than any other because the effectiveness of the delivery system is dependent upon such variables as setting, climate, abilities of nurses, desires and needs of the client, and beliefs and nursing philosophies of institutions.

Basically there are four systems for delivery of nursing care: (1) functional, (2) team, (3) case, and (4) primary care. But combinations of these methods with new modes for provision of service are evolving all the time. A nurse-leader is more apt to review the expected outcomes, that is, what one wishes to have occur as a result of a designated delivery system. Being goal oriented, the deliberator can develop a system for administration of care that will provide the desired product—continuous and comprehensive nursing care.

The *functional system* of care involves a method of work organization and personnel assignment in which tasks are divided and assigned to personnel in the interest of time and expediency of service. This mode of operation is the system most often utilized in nursing. Personnel are fittted into fixed slots; one person passes medications, another administers treatments, and others provide hygienic care or do simple tasks such as making beds. Still others may be assigned to such special tasks as helping at the desk by recording for staff and serving as liaison between patients, doctors, family members, and others concerned with the patients.

The task-centered approach to nursing care has been borrowed from industry, where mass production is desired and the assembly line system proves to be the most effective means for achieving goals. As in industry, there are situations and times in nursing when uniformity in work patterns and mass production of nursing services is desirable. In instances where there are many patients and few care givers, the work forces are of necessity assigned with the greatest attention to conservation of manpower. Another rationale might be that only one qualified person is available to perform specific tasks (to administer inhalation therapy or to teach a diabetic the administration of insulin), which limits the delegation of special assignments to one individual. Functional nursing is usually viewed by administrators as the most economical way to provide nursing services; however, to achieve true cost effectiveness many elements must be considered. Recognition of the needs of the client, attention to the satisfactions and dissatisfactions of the care givers, and the philosophy and goals of the providers of health services are to be weighed in the light of the selected system. Cost studies indicate other methods are as cost effective as, and sometimes are more so than, functional nursing care.

The *team system** is a mode developed in the 1950's for providing care in which a professional nurse facilitates the efforts of a group of diversified health care personnel to provide for the health needs of an individual or a group of people in either a hospital or a community setting. In team nursing the leader's primary responsibility is to see that every activity is characterized by mutual sharing and exploration based on an interest and concern for the individuals served. All efforts are directed toward accomplishing group tasks with as much efficiency and expediency as possible. The thrust of every activity is directed toward delivery of individualized health care. Through the team process the nurse-leader plans, participates in, coordinates, interprets, supervises, and evaluates the care given. Consistent and continuous high quality care is made possible through the development of written nursing care plans developed by the nurse-

---

*See also Douglass, L. M.: Review of team nursing, St. Louis, 1973, The C. V. Mosby Co., chap. 1.

leader and co-workers, with evaluation and revision of care plans as new insights are gained.

Team nursing is a philosophy, not simply a methodology. There is nothing new about the idea of assembling a cluster of people to work toward the solution of specific problems. The uniqueness of team nursing becomes apparent when the beliefs and values of the system are understood. The philosophy of team nursing subscribes to the worth of the individual, with priority given to those being served and to those delivering the service, to the need for a prepared person to be the overall coordinator and interpreter of plans for care, to functioning of members as coequals with minimal emphasis on hierarchical lines of demarcation between the leader and the led, and to a sensitivity and responsiveness to the need for adaptability and change.

To be effective the team plan for nursing requires that care givers be led by one qualified to practice leadership, that all team members be committed to the philosophy of team nursing, that all members possess knowledge and understanding inherent in their roles, that individual members and the group be technically skilled for their assignments, and that the members function collaboratively and cooperatively.

The *case system* is perhaps the oldest method of care delivery. It is used when one-to-one contact is desired. A single individual is assigned to one client where constant care and observation is desired for a specified period of time. In this system the nurse has the responsibility for total nursing care of the patient. In hospitals the case method is most commonly adopted for the care of acutely ill patients, such as those in intensive care units. The one-to-one mode is almost the standard method of assignment for student nurses. In the community the case system is practiced where individual contact is made by public health and mental health nurses. A nurse practitioner's case load can include as many clients as the care giver can handle effectively. There are situations when the client requires or desires seclusion or separation from the general public. In these instances one-to-one care is usually in practice round the clock. Private duty nurses fill most of these needs and are usually on call for service through a professional registry.

The *primary care system,* a concept of nursing care developed in 1968, embodies the principle that direct access of nurse to patient or client with the nurse accepting full responsibility for his own functioning and decisions produces a more effective method for delivery of nursing care and thus provides continuous quality care to the patient. The role of the primary nurse requires an ability to form therapeutic relationships with individuals, to make decisions and assume responsibility, to conduct interviews and obtain and assess pertinent data, and to communicate effectively with peers and members of other health care disciplines. The primary nurse has the total pervasive responsibility for planning and directing client care for 24 hours a day throughout the client's need or desire for primary nursing service. The primary nurse is held accountable for planning comprehensive care and for formulating clear-cut nursing directions for others to continue that care. Each primary nurse coordinates his own activities with clients, physicians, and other personnel. An associate nurse can be assigned to the care of a patient whose primary nurse is off duty. The relief nurse's function is to carry out the care plan designed by the primary nurse. The number of patients a primary nurse can care for depends on such variables as rapidity of patient turnover, the amount and kind of medical treatment and nursing services required, numbers of persons involved in client care, and the effectiveness and efficiency of the support services.

Primary care can be arranged by contractual agreement between client and nurse or between physician and nurse or can be practiced within the structure of an employing agency. Proponents of the primary nursing delivery system believe this model takes on a whole new concept of caring for a patient and that the individual competence level of each nurse is manifested in respect to performance as a nurse rather than as a manager of people.

All these systems designed for provision of nursing care have strengths and weaknesses that influence achievement of the goals of continuity and comprehensiveness of client care. Factors such as economics, communications, needs of clients, and needs of personnel are to be considered when a system for delivery of nursing care is selected.

PREDICTIVE PRINCIPLE: *Guidelines such as established channels, methods, and provision for communication within an agency enable the nurse-leader to delegate tasks and authority appropriately.*

PREDICTIVE PRINCIPLE: *Clear lines of communication promote morale among organization members and enhance goal accomplishment.*

Essential characteristics of an organization include communication and decision-making procedures. The effectiveness of an organization depends in part on its having the right information at the right place at the right time. In dealing with communication among individuals who are linked together to provide health care, one needs a model of the aspects of communication or a way to indicate the status of affairs in decision making. Communication in health agencies involves provision for (1) the patients and clients to communicate with each other, (2) nursing care givers to communicate with each other and with various health care disciplines, and (3) the hierarchy to communicate both horizontally and vertically.

Development of a communication model requires knowledge of (1) a communication network that exists at a given time, (2) knowledge of existing control processes in the agency (policies and procedures), and (3) knowledge of how existing agency and control process affect change.

Communication in administration involves provision for major responsibilities: channels, methods, and opportunities for (1) the hierarchy to communicate outward, (2) the line and staff to communicate with the hierarchy, (3) the personnel to communicate on interdepartmental levels, and (4) individual clients and nurse to communicate independently with each other.

Channels of communication utilized in the case and functional plans of nursing care are illustrated in Fig. 4. In these systems, assignment of care is made by the charge nurse. A major difference in the systems lies in the area of responsibility. In the case method a single care giver assumes responsibility for

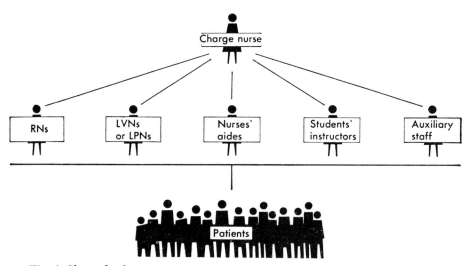

Fig. 4. Channels of communication in case and functional plans of nursing care.

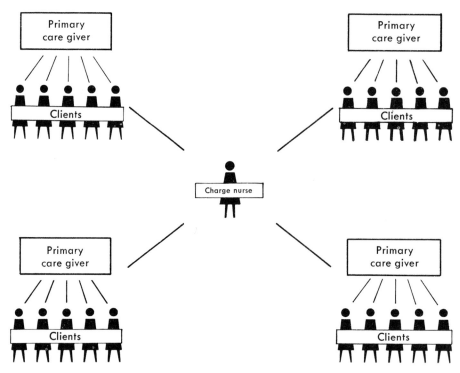

Fig. 5. Channels of communication in primary care nursing.

the total care of a patient, whereas in the functional method a group of task-oriented persons provide services collectively to a number of patients. In each method the charge nurse remains the authority figure through whom all major communications are channeled.

In the practice of primary care the line of communication (Fig. 5) lies more strongly between one care giver and one or more patients, depending on the variables in the situation. The care giver either chooses or is assigned by a nurse-leader to patients according to the clients' needs and wishes, the nurse's abilities, special interests, and expertise, or the work situation. The nurse assumes full responsibility for administering care to one or more patients and views other care givers and the charge nurse as resource persons for validation, suggestions, or assistance. In short, the primary care method incorporates a collegial relationship rather than operating in a hierarchical system.

When team nursing is employed, as illustrated in Fig. 6, channels of communication are established whereby the charge nurse delegates leadership responsibility to a nurse-leader for a group of patients. The team system provides the nurse-leader opportunity to employ any or all methods of assignment according to the assessed needs of the clients and the capabilities and desires of the care givers and receivers. Theoretically, because of the leader's strategic position in terms of influencing and implementing plans, he is influential in motivating personnel and in building a team that will achieve the aims of the group. In this system, team members relate to the nurse-leader, who in turn relates directly to the charge nurse. The charge nurse serves as a resource person and is freer to

Fig. 6. Channels of communication in team nursing.

engage in the promotion and maintenance of comprehensive and continuous care for the clients under the jurisdiction of the nursing teams.

PREDICTIVE PRINCIPLE: *Reactions to stress influence efficiency of performance in the work situation.*

Sickness in and of itself is stress producing, not only to the people who are ill but also to those persons who are giving care. Much of nursing still takes place around the sick individual or in critical situations. The critical nature of nursing practice provokes a high stress environment and engenders a great feeling of responsibility within the providers of nursing care. This of itself makes nursing care of people more vulnerable to additional stresses, which can occur either in the course of their personal lives or in interaction with their colleagues at work. Individuals develop patterns for coping with stress; similarly, groups that work together fall into set ways of dealing with stressful situations. These patterns may or may not be the best way of coping, but at least they allow the individual or group members to perform in the situation. For the individual nurse or group it is necessary to study and validate appropriate and applicable methods for handling critical situations that create stresses in the work program. The reader is referred to the work of Gwen Marram for an in depth study of leadership interventions in times of stress.*

INVESTMENT OF AUTHORITY

Authority can be given or assumed by an individual or group because of power of personality, position, knowledge, or ability. Authority and leadership have similar meanings. Both terms give formal managerial sanction to an individual or group. Leadership positions can be floating. The assumption of the leadership role carries with it responsibility and authority, whether formalized or not. There is *official* authority, which is invested in a group or a leader by the hierarchy or by the group one is working with, or both. Then there is *assumed* authority. Sometimes assumed leadership is stable, or it may move within the group, one individual at a time being the leader; at other times several individuals lead simultaneously. Difficulty arises only when two participants who have assumed authority are in conflict, resulting in a power struggle. Both official and assumed leadership roles are legitimate sources of authority.

To be effective a leader must be assured of the authority to carry out his directives within the employing agency. Effective delegation of authority in meeting the organizational objectives depends on the willingness of management to release decision-making powers to members within the institution and the willingness of those who are asked to lead to accept the leadership role with its inherent responsibilities and accountability. Finding the balance between too much and too little investment of authority promotes a management process that can be satisfying to the nurse-leader as well as to the participants.

PREDICTIVE PRINCIPLE: *The nurse-leader's belief that ultimate accountability lies with him determines the scope and limitations he sets for his leadership.*

---

*Marram, G. D.: The group approach in nursing practice, St. Louis, 1973, The C. V. Mosby Co.

Delegation of authority never relieves the leader of the basic responsibilities inherent in the position. The nurse-leader takes full responsibility for whatever actions occur as a result of his delegation of authority. Just as individual members are held accountable to their leader, so the leader is accountable to his immediate supervisor.

Once delegation of authority is made, each care giver will then be held accountable to the delegator. The nurse-leader has a responsibility for maintaining a continuing relationship with care givers to ensure that care is given with continuity, safety, and effectiveness.

ASSIGNMENT MAKING

Development of an assignment-making plan may be rational, deliberative, habitual, purposeful, or random, or any combination of these, depending on the knowledge, experience, and skill of the leader. In the case method, assignments change from shift to shift and often from day to day or from week to week and are delegated usually by territory. For example, the nurse is directed to take one patient in room 419 or to care for three patients in rooms 420 and 421. In the functional method, assignments are delegated by the tasks to be completed. For example, one is instructed to make beds, and another to pass medications. In the team system, groups are divided by territory, and within that territory, assignments are made according to difficulty of patient care and the preparation and/or the abilities of the nurse in combination often with territory. These assignments also tend to change at least weekly.

Primary nursing has no territory. In this system the care giver either chooses or is assigned by a nurse-leader to patients according to the client's needs and wishes and the nurse's abilities and special interests, specific areas, and expertise, as well as according to the individual case load. All care is planned on a 24-hour basis and on the nurse's working with the patient for the duration of his stay in the hospital and sometimes during his return if it is anticipated. In some conditions, plans include continuing client care into the home.

PREDICTIVE PRINCIPLE: *A thorough problem-oriented approach to patient-centered care enables the care giver to develop effective nursing care plans for the client or patient.*

Once authority is delegated, the recipient has the responsibility for carrying through the tasks assigned. Part of the care giver's responsibility can be met through assessment of the institution, determination of the client's needs, and the development of viable care plans, all of which is an integral part of the decentralization of nursing responsibilities. Fay Bower, in *The Process of Planning Nursing Care* outlines four phases of planning nursing care: (1) assessment, (2) problem identification, (3) formulation of plans for nursing action, and (4) planning for evaluation.*

---

*Bower, F. L.: The process of planning nursing care: a theoretical model, St. Louis, 1972, The C. V. Mosby Co., chap. 1.

PREDICTIVE PRINCIPLE: *Assignment of authority necessitates a willingness on the part of the nurse-leader to relinquish authority.*

The leader who feels secure in his knowledge and ability can develop a behavior pattern and promote an atmosphere that will allow responsible participants to function on a dependent-interdependent relationship with support from the leader. This in no way abridges the nurse's role as leader. The leader still controls the operation in an atmosphere acceptable to everyone. Trust is established, and members are encouraged to develop their capabilities to their maximum potential within the limitations of the job. The leader is concerned about control so that quality is maintained. There are ways to ensure quality of care without restricting the care giver in such a manner that his authority and responsibility are weakened or usurped. By serving as a validator and a quality control individual, the nurse-leader (1) is available, (2) makes suggestions, and (3) establishes a peer relationship with the care giver. As a resource person and consultant, the nurse-leader makes relinquishing of authority more realistic and easier.

PREDICTIVE PRINCIPLE: *A sufficient number of prepared personnel allows effective delegation of authority to meet organizational and patient needs.*

PREDICTIVE PRINCIPLE: *Matching the abilities of care givers to the jobs to be done increases work productivity and individual job satisfaction.*

Administration usually controls the number of workers assigned to any unit. Health agencies determine the categories and numbers of personnel required to maintain their institutions. They seek to maintain a stable nurse-patient ratio that will ensure the implementation of safe, problem-oriented care. It is obvious that patients with many and varied needs require more nursing services than those who have relatively few problems.

The delegator is allotted a number of care givers according to the number of personnel available for the work period. It is the nurse-leader's task to assign the members so that the best interests of the patients, staff, and agency are realized.

The leader, for example, may have a client who is placed in reverse isolation and who exhibits many feelings of insecurity. The nurse-leader has three care givers who can practice reverse isolation safely. The leader reasons that one nurse is new to the agency and therefore somewhat insecure; a second is technically skillful but is inclined to be abrupt in the initial approach to patients. A third nurse is capable of caring for physical needs and is problem oriented in relationships with patients. The leader will, of course, choose the latter of the three to care for the patient, realizing the best interests of patient, staff, and agency will be served.

Note should be taken that the primary nurse may also stipulate care either to the family or to the patient himself; usually the practitioner decides in collaboration with the client what is to be done and to whom it will be delegated.

The delegator who knows both the qualifications required for the jobs in the health agency and the abilities and personalities of the care givers is better able to utilize each person's capabilities productively and maximally. In any organizational structure, however, personnel factors do not remain constant. Frequently the nurse-leader is assigned a member who is new to the situation and sometimes to the nursing profession. Even if the orientation to the agency is complete and the in-service program extensive, the new employee will require assistance and close supervision from the nurse-leader to allow for assessment of his capabilities and appropriate delegation of assignment.

Assigning uncomplicated tasks to a beginner increases his self-confidence and facilitates his progress. The worker should be encouraged to learn and increase his skills, with emphasis on his strengths, so that learning the art of administering quality patient care can be accelerated. Gradually increasing the difficulty of jobs assigned, within job specifications, promotes increased feelings of responsibility and worth and results in optimum productivity.

The nurse-leader can accomplish these tasks, however, only when qualified persons are available in sufficient number. When this is not so, the leader must compromise the assignment. The patient must be kept as the focal point, and only his priority needs are met. The charge nurse should be alerted and should take steps to increase the staff to the necessary number.

Because of the number of variables associated with administration of care, there is no definitive statement of optimal nurse-patient ratio. One trend in nursing is that the RN-LVN-aide ratio is becoming more expanded. In some places as salaries for nursing services increase, fewer RNs are being employed, and LVNs and aides are hired as replacements. Professional nurses have a responsibility to determine the RN-patient ratio they believe necessary for the administration of safe, problem-oriented client care and then work for the maintenance of that essential ratio. In determining the number of personnel needed, close examination should be given to the various systems of care delivery available. For example, in the team plan, where team leaders are assigned to groups of workers, the supervisory staff is pyramided, thus removing them from the care-giving role. In primary care, more persons are actually giving basic nursing care, making this system more cost effective in the final analysis. Studies are in progress to determine whether nurses' aides are actually cost effective. Because of their limited abilities in some care delivery systems, such as primary care, aides are not considered cost effective. In light of these investigations, some institutions have begun altering their staffing patterns. One way this is being done is by replacing aides with LVNs and RNs as the number of aides decreases through attrition.

PREDICTIVE PRINCIPLE: *Centralization of information storage and information giving and retrieval systems allows for efficient assessment, delegation, and implementation of tasks.*

The care giver is in a key position to obtain and store information concerning the client. A variety of sources are tapped for information. Records, reports, orders, and messages—both written and verbal—provide input for processing information. People are not as efficient nor as effective with storage and retrieval of information as machines. For this reason many nursing units are incorporating mechanical devices to facilitate the care-giving process. The cassette tape recorder is one medium widely used for transcribing messages and activities. Individual care givers condense their reports to pertinent issues and record them as they have time. The nurse or group coming to the work scene listens to the tape while the worker or group going off completes their assignment. If there is need for clarification or additional information, reporting personnel are accessible for dialogue. New persons who need filling in on detail seek out the care giver after he has read the patient's record and appraised himself of the situation.

Computers are a major mode of storing information centrally. These technical devices are in operation in many health agencies and will become a common adjunct to most nursing arenas within the next few years. An individual can feed the client's identifying data into the system and can receive whatever information concerning the client that is needed to facilitate the practice of nursing.

PREDICTIVE PRINCIPLE: *Clear and concise directions enhance task delegation.*

Assignments for care givers should be both written and verbal. Definite plans should be devised to impart information. Members need to know such specifics as whom they will be caring for, where the patients are located, special tasks, coffee and lunch breaks, and any additional commitment. Assignments should be posted in an area easily accessible to staff members and early enough to allow the personnel time to arrange individual schedules. Verbal directions can be given through prerecordings, on a one-to-one basis, or in a conference held early in the work period.

Members function better when they know the extent of their assignment. Leaders who withhold part of the work assignment to spare the worker the pain of hearing a large assignment or who believe that delegating a task little by little is better than making one large assignment are operating on false assumptions. Members need to know what demands will be made of them to make the best use of their time. Assignments differ when primary care is in progress in that the care givers often arrange their time and tasks around the needs of the client with a central arrangement for relief.

PREDICTIVE PRINCIPLE: *A balance between variety and consistency of assignment increases worker's motivation and productivity.*

Ideally, a member should be given the same patient assignment at least from one day off until the next. Studies are showing that assigning primary responsibility for a care giver for the duration of the client's stay is more rewarding to the patient and the nurse and ensures the client of better care since there is more opportunity to know the patient and to administer quality care on a continuous basis. The only times the client-nurse relationship should be broken are when the nurse and patient have some basic inability to get along, when the care giver finds he cannot meet the patient's needs, or when the nurse has time off. Consistency with assignment allows the worker time to become familiar with the patients and members of the nursing staff. It is well to rotate members from one geographic setting to another to ensure continued flexibility within the department. Occasionally, delegators receive requests from members to remain with the same group or in the same location for long periods of time with such statements as, "I'm more comfortable on the east side," or "I work better with Miss Judd and Mrs. Sampson." Astute leaders will recognize participants' emotional needs but will work with the members to help them understand and accept the rationale of assignments.

Tasks assigned to members are best completed if they are palatable and stimulating. "The work isn't hard," one nurses' aide observed, "It's the never ending monotony of the job." Routinization is often favored in an effort to facilitate getting the job done and to conserve expense. Too much sameness reduces the degree to which an individual can participate in the organization affairs of his work and often prevents him from completing a task that is meaningful to him. A nurse assigned to giving preoperative medications day after day and week after week will lose the opportunity to experience the broader implications of nursing care.

If the delegator varies the member's assignments over a period of time to include the total spectrum of care, the member will grow and develop the ability to employ diverse physical, cognitive, and interpersonal skills. In addition, a limited assignment is not economically beneficial to an agency because the employee's training and potential are not being realized.

PREDICTIVE PRINCIPLE: *Consideration for each care giver's preferences and areas of expertise influences morale.*

Giving thought to members' choices of one assignment over another fosters job satisfaction. Nothing makes a person feel so good about himself as having success in what he is doing; one way to assure success is to delegate assignments according to the care giver's preferences and expertise, matching these with the needs of the client. Factors that have a bearing on the care giver's preference of assignment include (1) physical characteristics of the job (such as the extent of walking, lifting, and standing) and the type of physical activity involved (such as hygienic care or working with specialized equipment), (2) the degree of independence permitted, (3) the fairness with which the member feels he is being treated, (4) whether he has had a part in policy and procedure making, (5) individual commitment to the decisions, and (6) the degree to which the assignment interests him.

Information concerning preferences should be acquired in a professional and systematic manner to assure each member equal consideration. The nurse-leader can learn the desires of employees through observation, conferences, and evaluation. Knowledge of a worker's preference for a task does not imply that the member will be given priority. It may be that two or more members wish the same assignment, or an individual may express a desire to engage in work he is incapable of performing. Another may request an assignment in which he excels, not wishing to extend his experience beyond that which he knows to be satisfying. The nurse-leader will consider the wishes of all members and make assignments in the best interests of the patient, personnel, and agency.

PREDICTIVE PRINCIPLE: *A systematic planning process predisposes effective delegation.*

One prime quality the nurse-leader must have to delegate assignments effectively is the ability to examine and deal with ever changing situations. The ability to see problems and issues is not an innate quality. Such insights are cultivated and require consistent practice in uncovering significant facts, in weighing evidence, foreseeing contingencies, developing alternatives, and finding the best person for the care to be given.

The delegator can utilize several approaches. He can follow past procedure, observe and copy others, adhere strictly to rules and regulations, adopt the scientific method, or use any combination of these methods.

To model assignments after those methods that have been utilized in the past is static. The follower of standard routines seldom investigates the "why" of an assignment and has little concern with new techniques. "It's always been done this way," provides a satisfactory explanation for the practice in question. For example, in the past a common practice in assigning tasks to others was to determine the number of personnel available for a given day and to divide this figure into the total number of patients to be cared for, with no regard for the patients' individual and priority needs or the workers' capacity to meet them. Such a practice usually leads to casual reorganization of labor by the staff members involved in an effort to correct the inequities of assignment; chaos results.

Another approach to learning the methodology of assignment is through observation and discussion with other nurse-leaders in similar situations. The leader selects for his own use what is believed to be the best of his fellow leaders' techniques for coordinating group activities. Exchange of experiences among nurse-leaders is common practice and can contribute to the improvement of managerial technique, especially if the leader has the opportunity to participate in workshops and institutes that include representatives from a variety of situations. Most leaders enjoy discussing their methods and tend to speak of those experiences and practices in which they are successful. There is an element of danger in attempting to apply one leader's methods to another situation, however. A practice that works well for one leader might produce poor results for a person who copies it. Ineffectiveness of the adapted method can be attributed to such variables as differences in goals, personnel, size of department, and the composition of nursing groups. Such sharing of experiences, if used as the only source of information, may limit the leader's knowledge and narrow perspective, thus failing to develop the full potential of the nursing delegator's abilities.

A third plan for work distribution is to strictly follow the directives of the agency by adhering to job descriptions, policies, and procedures without concern for individual differences. This manner of delegating keeps the assignments fettered, develops rigid habits for handling work assignments, and prevents the development of flexible attitudes and the full utilization of people.

Adaptation of methodology much like the scientific method of delegation of responsibility is evolving a logical approach for the nurse-leader. The basic mechanism of the scientific method is to create and test a plan and to evaluate its effectiveness, after which conclusions may be drawn. In pure science a body of knowledge is obtained by means of experiments conducted to confirm or disprove the proposition under consideration. The hypothesis is tested under carefully controlled conditions. During the experiments, observations are made and data kept to record what has happened, when, and how. Classifications are made, and interpretations and generalizations are drawn. The outcome of such studies may be the formation of a basic law or principle indicating that when certain activities take place under stated conditions, the results will be of a specific sort.

Scientific knowledge about the management of personnel cannot be considered in the same sense as are the pure sciences because of the variables in individuals and their personal social structures. There is, however, a body of knowledge in the field of management from which general principles have been developed. It is feasible and practiceable to adapt the methods used in the scientific process to delegate responsibility in nursing, but utilization of the problem-solving approach requires that the nurse-leader have a clear understanding of the steps to be taken.

The first prerequisite to coordinated effort is a goal. The overall objective of any group engaged in service is to achieve maximum operational effectiveness in reaching goals. Activity programmed for success leads to accomplishment of goals and results in an awareness of and a mutual expression of a sense of fulfillment. The delegator of responsibility observes and analyzes the situation within the context of responsibility to determine what is to be accomplished in a given period of time.

An American Nurses' Association position paper describes the components of nursing as caring, curing, and coordinating.* This definition clearly places responsibility on the nurse for activities other than those usually thought of as patient centered. In this broader definition of care, nurse-leaders formulate goals to include (1) the needs of the client (preventive, sustaining, curative, or rehabilitative care), (2) provision for smooth coordination of services (attention to timing when administering care, avoidance of overlap of duties, planning with others for coverage during lunch and coffee break and conference times, being certain that routine tasks are appropriated, providing coverage for possible emergencies or unusual circumstances), (3) consideration of the capabilities, limitations, needs, and desires of personnel, and (4) collaboration with others of the health care team.

When the problems and goals are identified, an assignment can be made. At this stage, knowledge, insight, imagination, intuition, and experience are brought to bear to construct a plan that will meet the needs of the situation under consideration. This process involves assessment, problem identification formulating plans for nursing action, planning for evaluation, and implementation.†

The plan is then observed in action and analyzed. It must be evaluated in terms of the objectives and subsequent activity. The variables are measured by the nurse as they operate in the situation (work completed on time, overlap of activities, appreciative patient, discontented staff member, handling of emer-

---

*Educational preparation for nurse practitioners and assistants to nurses: a position paper, New York, 1965, American Nurses Association, p. 5.
†Bower, F. L.: The process of planning nursing care: a theoretical model, St. Louis, 1972, The C. V. Mosby Co., chap. 1.

gency situation). If the nurse-leader establishes that methods of assignment allow the nurses to achieve the goals they have set, there is reason to believe the methods used were valid and can be employed again with assurance. If, on the other hand, it is discovered that the methods of assignment led to undesirable results, the nurse-leader should review the methods employed and establish at which point in the process ineffectiveness began and trouble or failure occurred. The leader will then determine who was involved, what the circumstances were, and when, where, and why the breakdown occurred. He will then go back and rework the method at the point of failure to improve the procedure.

MEASURING RESULTS

The evaluation process in nursing is the establishment of the value of operational actions by weighing them in relationship to, for example, established criteria specific to the goals of an agency or delegator, to care giver's performance or patient care (as are behavioral objectives), or "norms" such as expected or usual outcomes. The evaluation process is a comparison of something to something. The primary purpose for nursing evaluation is to determine if the nursing action met the goal, if it can be repeated, or if another action needs to be considered. Nursing care is a self-corrective system, rather like an equilateral triangle with three fixed points of plan: (1) operation, (2) reaction, and (3) evaluation, each feeding into the other and each moving from one to the other with fluidity. Without evaluation, operations and the people enacting those operations do not improve.

Roles involved in the evaluation process include the evaluator, the evaluated, and the receiver of the evaluation. (The reader is referred to Chapters 1 and 5 for more detail.) It is possible for one person to engage in all these roles, seeking validation from another person.

PREDICTIVE PRINCIPLE: *Assignments that have clearly defined standards and goals provide a basis for measurement of outcome.*

The nurse-leader is interested in measuring a diversity of activities within a given assignment. He wants to be sure that individual and group output is of satisfactory quality and quantity and is completed within the prescribed time. The leader desires that resources, people, plant, and equipment are used to the best advantage and that patients receive the full benefit of services. Clearly delineated guidelines are necessary for the evaluation process to function effectively. Guidelines provide an orderly procedure for planning and assessing the caliber and degree of support for health care and for providing institutional services and nursing activities.

Another dimension of the evaluation process is assessment of the contractual agreement. The making of a contract, whether it be verbal or written, has become an important mode of attaining goals. In lieu of the nurse-leader's delegating specific assignments to personnel, as is the case in the functional or team systems of care, the care giver (examples are the primary care giver or one who is engaged in a special assignment, such as teaching) enters into a contract with the client, with another nurse, or with some other person to carry out the agreement for reaching a specific goal or goals in a specified length of time. The contractual agreement is exemplified in the situation in which a client (the led) and the nurse (the leader) contract with each other for a given amount of instruction in the irrigation and dressing of the patient's leg wound.

The collaborators divide the tasks into realistic stages of accomplishment, using criteria based on quality of performance but keeping in mind that time limits must remain flexible, for health crises do not lend themselves to rigid time schedules. For example, in the first stage the client will observe the nurse in the entire nursing procedure while engaging in purposeful dialogue about it (that is, how, when, where, what, and why). The patient will read information pertinent to the procedure, supplied by the nurse. In the second stage, with nurse supervision, the client will prepare the necessary equipment for irrigation and will remove his dressings, doing both without contamination. He validates actions and understanding with criteria listed in procedure manual and with his nurse. The third stage will be realized in the client's performance of the wound irrigation. He continues to follow designated procedure (accurate temperature and adequate strength of solution, direction of flow, protection of linens from drainage). In the fourth and final stage the client will learn from the nurse the art of applying a sterile dressing. He opens dressing without contamination, applies it directly to the wound with sure movement, and fixes it firmly in place with adhesive or bandage.

By such specific agreement and mutual acceptance of responsibility, criteria are established, making the outcomes of this alternative mode as measurable as those within the more traditional systems of care.

Both leader and led must be aware of the goals for the day and must know exactly what is expected of them in terms of quantity, quality, and time if they are to be held responsible members for attaining goals. Assignments, leader-participant contact, and group conferences, coupled with accessibility of resource people and necessary information, will give the required criteria and data for measuring results.

One cannot discuss assessment of goal achievement without speaking of mastery of the goal. In some instances there is room for degree of accomplishment, as in the process of bed making, in learning an unsterile technique, or in various levels of communication. At other times, no latitude can be allowed. Any break in sterile technique is untenable. Inappropriate counsel or action in crisis intervention may lead to disaster. The nurse-leader builds in the criteria all the contingencies necessary for desired practice and assesses outcomes accordingly. With a clear delineation in the nurse's role then nurse-leader can become the facilitator, validator, collaborator, resource person, and consultant. In this way the leader applies his managerial skills largely to direct client care and is interested in said care and in the growing ability of people to provide such service rather than using these skills to meet the logistical requirements of management. However, the nurse-leader does retain the ability and authority to delegate those logistics to another person because logistics and direct client care are interwoven and do influence each other.

Some leaders believe they must check personally on all details of an assignment if control of assignments is to be maintained. This autocratic manager feels confident only when he has witnessed the completion of his directions. Such restrictive measures usually result in (1) employee expectation of close supervision, (2) generation of subservient feelings, (3) exhibition of routine, compliant behavior patterns, and (4) lack of assumption of responsibility for the worker's own actions.

The effective leader will find it not only impossible but also undesirable to review personally all aspects of performance and consequently must select certain critical points that will provide an adequate indication of what is going on. In developing the checking process the leader must take into consideration expenditure of time as well as employee reaction to the evaluative process.

In nursing operation the leader assumes responsibility for the overall functions but in the process of assignment making will delegate the duty of checking certain functions to care givers who are capable of assuming the role. Responsibility for review of progress can be on an individual basis or may be extended to several members. For example, an experienced member may be given four patients to care for on a primary care basis. The member learns the major needs of the patients and is given freedom to devise his own care plan and schedule for the day.

Another avenue of sharing responsibility for measurement of results is through group effort. The nurse-leader, for instance, may have been informed by group members of a belief that there is wasted effort in each worker's having to interrupt his individual patient assignment to run errands, such as transporting patients, calling for late trays, and locating special pieces of equipment. The delegator could request all care givers to engage in a measuring procedure over a specific period of time to learn who was interrupted, for what purpose, and the frequency of interruption. The group could then study the results of the survey to develop a design for greater efficiency. The reader is referred to Chapter 5 more more explicit information concerning the evaluation process.

PREDICTIVE PRINCIPLE: *Frequent comparison of actual performance with criteria determines the quality of care and the level of actual performance.*

Accurate identification and documentation of behaviors of members practicing nursing is most difficult. The problem of measurement of clinical competence is compounded because of (1) the variety of clinical problems encountered by the nurse, (2) the number of methods employed to deal with these problems, (3) the paucity of significant and useful research to validate the utilization of one methodology over another, (4) the difficulty of directly observing all activities, and (5) the tendency on the part of individuals to describe behavior in terms of their beliefs and principles, which may or may not bear relation to reality.

If tasks have been clearly defined and recorded, it should be a relatively easy matter to identify the people concerned with the activities. Similarly, if a predetermined time schedule of operation has been formulated, the leader can ascertain the level of progress at any specific time within the work period. It is reasonable to assume then, that the nurse-leader will have an overall understanding of the entire operation at all times.

The evaluator's task is very often complicated by the blurred role of the nurse-leader. Managerial skills can be divided into two classifications, those that are concrete or specific and those that are abstract or rather indefinite. Concrete managerial level skills, such as manipulating task-oriented activities, making sure enough equipment and supplies are available for the care givers to use, and other logistic activities, are fairly easily accomplished. Abstract managerial skills, usually having to do with interpersonal relationships, are much less easily defined and less easily delegated. As nursing becomes able to sort out technical aspects and to delegate these to ward clerks, unit managers, or other business-oriented people, it will be better able to focus on the comparative aspects of performance relative to assignment.

APPLICATION OF PREDICTIVE PRINCIPLES IN THE DELEGATION OF AUTHORITY

As the nurse-leader, you are responsible for planning and directing the work being done on the unit. You have made the work assignments for the day, and an LVN comes to you with the following statement: "I have had the same assignment for three weeks, and I am tired of it. I would like to learn how to assist with the debridement of burns treatment for Johnny."

PROBLEM	PREDICTIVE PRINCIPLES	PRESCRIPTION
The LVN is dissatisfied with the work assignment and wishes to increase in knowledge and skills.	Clear lines of communication promote morale among organization members and enhance goal accomplishment.	Encourage LVN to express feelings by listening and giving encouraging motions and words.
	Understanding the categories and roles of nursing personnel enables the delegator to select the type and number of personnel appropriate for the job.	Confirm with LVN that request is legitimate and that the assignment for the day will be unchanged but that plans will be made for change.
	A balance between variety and consistency of assignment increases worker's motivation and productivity.	
	Written descriptions of policies, procedures, and/or guidelines by which an employee may handle situations when they occur promote ease of operation for the care giver and control of the authority delegated by the nurse-leader.	Help LVN locate material and resources that will prepare her for the learning episode, e.g., procedure manual, books, nurse.
	Matching the abilities of care givers to the jobs to be done increases work productivity and individual job satisfaction.	Schedule LVN to assist in the care of the burn patient. Arrange for double coverage until LVN is competent.
	Clear and concise directions enhance task delegation.	Inform LVN when and with whom she will be working.

Continued.

PROBLEM	PREDICTIVE PRINCIPLES	PRESCRIPTION
Dissatisfaction with assignment—cont'd	Assignment of authority necessitates a willingness on the part of the nurse-leader to relinquish authority.	Trust LVN to fulfill responsibilities.
	Assignments that have clearly defined standards and goals provide a basis for measurement of outcome. Frequent comparison of actual performance with criteria determines the quality of care and the level of actual performance.	Observe procedure periodically and at strategic times. Obtain feedback from patient, nurse-teacher, physician, and LVN.
	Consideration for each care giver's preferences and areas of expertise influences morale.	Be observant for other interests and expertise of LVN. Build into future assignments opportunities for variation.

BIBLIOGRAPHY

BOOKS

Argyris, C.: Management and organizational development, New York, 1971, McGraw-Hill Book Co.

Ayer, R.: Nursing service in transition: a description of organization for classification and utilization of nurse practitioners, Duarte, Calif., 1972, City of Hope Medical Center.

Berne, E.: Structure and dynamics of organizations and groups, Philadelphia, 1963, J. B. Lippincott Co.

Brown, E. L.: Newer dimensions of patient care. Part I. New York, 1961, Russell Sage Foundation.

Department of Health, Education, and Welfare, Secretary's Committee to Study Extended Roles for Nurses: Extending the scope of nursing practice, Washington, D.C., 1971, U.S. Government Printing Office.

French, W.: Personnel management process: human resources administration, ed. 2, Boston, 1970, Houghton Mifflin Co.

Lewis, E. P.: Changing patterns of nursing practice: new needs, new roles, New York, 1971, The American Journal of Nursing Co.

Likert, R.: New patterns in management, New York, 1961, McGraw-Hill Book Co.

Litterer, J. A.: Organizations, systems, control and adaptation, ed. 2, vol. 2, New York, 1969, John Wiley & Sons, Inc.

Lysaught, J. P., editor: National Commission for the Study of Nursing and Nursing Education: an abstract for action, New York, 1970, McGraw-Hill Book Co.

Mann, F. C., Indik, B., and Vroom, V.: The productivity of work groups, Ann Arbor,

Mich., 1963, Institute for social research, The University of Michigan Press.

National Institutes of Health: Planning for nursing needs and resources, Bethesda, April, 1972, Public Health Service no. 1741-0026, U.S. Department of Health, Education, and Welfare.

Tannenbaum, R., and Weschler, I. D.: Leadership and organization, a behavioral science approach, New York, 1961, McGraw-Hill Book Co.

Taylor, C.: In horizontal orbit, hospitals and cult of efficiency, New York, 1970, Holt, Rinehart and Winston, Inc.

PERIODICALS

Aydelotte, M.: Standard I, staffing for quality care, J. Nurs. Admin. pp. 33-36, March-April, 1973.

Chopra, A.: Motivation in task oriented groups, J. Nurs. Admin. pp. 55-60, Feb.-March, 1973.

Cononi, G. A., and Siler, M.: Automated multiphasic health testing in the hospital setting, J. Nurs. Admin. pp. 70-80, Nov.-Dec., 1972.

Department of Health, Education, and Welfare, Secretary's Committee to Study Extended Roles for Nurses: Extending the scope of nursing practice, Am. J. Nurs. 71(12): 2346-2351, 1971.

Department of Health, Education, and Welfare, Secretary's Committee to Study Extended Roles for Nurses: Extending the scope of nursing practice, Nurs. Outlook 20(1):46-52, 1972.

Fielding, V. V.: New team plan frees nurse, Mod. Hosp. 108(5):122-124, 1967.

Fry, W. F., and Lauer, J.: The planning team: why include nursing, leadership? J. Nurs. Admin. pp. 70-78, May, 1972.

Graves, H. H.: Can nursing shed bureaucracy? Am. J. Nurs. 71(3):491-494, 1971.

Hilgar, E. E.: Unit management systems, J. Nurs. Admin. pp. 43-49, Jan.-Feb., 1972.

Howe, G. E.: Decentralization aids coordination of patient care services, Hospitals 43:53-55, March, 1969.

Johnson, N. D.: The professional-bureaucratic conflict, J. Nurs. Admin. pp. 31-39, May-June, 1971.

Kinlein, M. L.: Independent nurse practitioner, Nurs. Outlook 20(1):22-23, 1972.

Knecht, A. A.: Innovation on four tower west/why? Am. J. Nurs. 73(5):809-810, 1973.

Manthey, M.: Primary care is alive and well in the hospital, Am. J. Nurs. 73(1):83-87, 1973.

Manthey, M., and Kramer, M.: A dialogue on primary nursing, Nurs. Forum 9(4):356-379, 1970.

Manthey, M., Ciske, K., Robertson, P., et al.: Primary nursing, Nurs. Forum 9(1):65-83, 1970.

Miller, D. I.: Standard II: organization is a process, J. Nurs. Admin. pp. 19-24, March-April, 1972.

Murray, D. L.: A case for independent group nursing practice, Nurs. Outlook 20(1):60-62, 1972.

Norris, C. M.: Direct access to the patient, Am. J. Nurs.70(5):1006-1010, 1970.

Schlegel, M. W.: Innovation on four tower west/how? Am. J. Nurs. 73(5):811-816, 1973.

Schwier, M. E., and Gardella, F. A.: Identifying the need for change in nursing service. Part I. Nurs. Outlook 18(4):56-62, 1970.

Sjarupa, J. A.: Management by objectives: a systematic way to manage change, J. Nurs. Admin. pp. 52-56, March-April, 1971.

Smith, M. L.: The clinical specialist: her role in staff development, J. Nurs. Admin. pp. 33-44, Jan.-Feb., 1971.

Somers, J. B.: A computerized nursing care system, Hospitals 45:93-100, April, 1971.

Stevens, B.: Analysis of trends in nursing care management, J. Nurs. Admin. pp. 12-17, Nov.-Dec., 1972.

White, H. C.: Some perceived behavior and attitudes of hospital employees under effective and ineffective supervisors, J. Nurs. Admin. pp. 49-54, Jan.-Feb., 1971.

White, M. B.: Importance of selected nursing activities, Nurs. Res. 21:4-14, Jan.-Feb., 1972.

CHAPTER FIVE

Predictive principles for evaluation

COMMITMENT OF ALL CONCERNED

Involvement of personnel in all phases of the evaluatory process increases belief in the fairness and accuracy of the evaluation, establishes a commitment to the evaluation, and increases motivation to utilize the results.

STANDARDS OF PRACTICE AND CRITERIA OF EVALUATION

Clear and concise role delineation and job descriptions enable employee, employer, and client to know the duties and responsibilities of the job.

Standards of performance and clear criteria for measuring performance increase the objectivity and validity of evaluation.

Evaluation of individual and small group activity necessitates establishment of criteria for the evaluation process.

A contract meeting enables the accountable nurse and the client to determine whether the contract has been met.

Use of appropriate assessment tools and sufficient evaluative data gathered from varied situations increases the validity of the conclusions.

Use of the self-evaluation process promotes growth and development of the appraiser and contributes to better quality of care.

Participation of patient or client in the evaluation of care contributes to an accurate and composite assessment.

A limited number of observations on an incidental basis jeopardizes the accuracy of evaluations.

Informal and formal assessments that are noted and recorded systematically provide significant input to the evaluation process.

Valid interpretation of data depends upon equitable evaluation of input.

The evaluator who establishes mutual trust and confidence with the evaluatee and who is familiar with the criteria of evaluation increases the accuracy and usefulness of the evaluation.

The degree to which the value systems of the evaluator and the evaluatee coincide influences their interpersonal relationships and directly affects the evaluation process.

DISPOSITIONAL ACTIVITIES

Frequent feedback on performance by a qualified evaluator, based on appropriate observations, reinforces desired behaviors and increases awareness of areas that need improvement.

Negative evaluative feedback accompanied with suggestions for improvement helps the evaluatee to change his behavior to more acceptable levels of performance.

An evaluation process that includes reciprocal participation both vertically and horizontally provides an avenue for high level morale and job satisfaction.

Evaluation is inherent in all categories of nursing activities and is discussed in each chapter as appropriate. Evaluation is a means to ascertain or appraise the value or amount of something in relationship to specific, desired outcomes, or goals. These expectations are either in the form of established criteria or expected outcomes specific to a health agency, care giver or client.

Traditionally the tendency has been to apply the evaluation procedure sporadically rather than continuously, by outside pressure rather than from within the system, for expediency rather than as an expression of planning, and after the fact rather than as part of preplanned, cumulative, and integrated design. Furthermore, nurses tend to restrict their evaluative views to themselves and to the small functional areas in which nursing care is implemented. Quality control among nurse practitioners is highly significant, but evaluation of other factors, such as agency procedures, organization structure, record forms, and personnel policies, are of equal importance. Larger units of the health care delivery system, such as the governing board and administration offering institutional services, must provide opportunity periodically and on an equal representation basis for reciprocal evaluation. When this happens, performance of nursing personnel is brought into proper focus and perspective.

The focus of this chapter is the evaluation of the nursing care giver; the overall purpose of evaluation is to assist the health organization, group, or individual member (care giver or client) to (1) determine the progress made toward achieving goals, (2) recognize and further develop strengths, (3) minimize weaknesses, (4) provide opportunity to demonstrate to assessors that worthiness exists, (5) develop more reliable instruments for assessment, and to (6) provide safety for the patient, personnel, agency, and community.

The fact that evaluation is a process implies that it involves a series of steps. Evaluation is one component of the problem-solving process and, as such, is part of the everyday nursing practice. There are a number of variables that can be used in an evaluative profile, and great differences of opinion exist as to their validity. Of importance is the nurse's progress with the assignment as it relates to (1) specific tasks and work responsibilities, (2) organizational resources, (3) observations, and (4) professional judgment by the person being appraised and the appraiser. Other vital input to the evaluation process is "third-party input," such as the assessments, views, opinions, and reactions of others whom the worker may encounter. Contacts with clients or patients, families, and other personnel can all provide relevant data.

Evaluation implies a reciprocal process. Organizational theorists affirm the problem of reciprocal evaluation to be one of determining effectiveness, that is, assessing whether the objectives or purposes of the system in process have been attained efficiently. Reciprocal appraisal is a way of saying that assessment has to take place in the context of the circumstances under which the nurse operates, with responsibility for nursing progress being shared by the determiners of those circumstances, including the patient. Accountability rests with all who participate in planning for and providing nursing care. If the hospital requests a tax override or bond issue, the community may choose to defeat it. This is an indicator or evaluative data about community support. If the nursing supervisor or head nurse asks agency administrators for necessary equipment and supplies, the administrators may or may not approve the purchase, which in turn may be an indicator or evaluator of the administrators' support. The nurse-leader may present a well-supported request for an additional staff member to help implement group responsibilities but may or may not have the request sanctioned. This is an indication for evaluation of the administration's responsiveness to nursing needs. The care giver may plan with a client for primary care. The degree to which the client cooperates with the implementation of that care is evaluative data about his commitment to the plan.

Traditionally in nursing, evaluation has been associated with unpleasant experiences during student days when the threat of failure was ever present. Judgments were all too often made with no help given to remedy actions under criticism, leaving the recipient feeling nervous and confused.

Confusion of evaluation with establishing a grade and the negative experiences most nurses have had with activities called "evaluation" have given this device a distasteful aura that is difficult to alter. Some agencies have modified the terminology used to remove negative connotations from the process. The evaluative procedure is sometimes referred to as "efficiency ratings," "performance assessment," and "appraisal." Whatever the term, all nurses evaluate, consciously or unconsciously, and the more knowledgeable nurse-leaders are about what evaluation is and how to evaluate, the more effective will be the use of this tool for improving patient care.

COMMITMENT OF ALL CONCERNED

Commitment means the act of pledging or binding oneself to a certain course or acts. Commitment first requires a conscious choice among alternatives, then a belief in the ideals that spawned that choice, and finally behaviors that actualize the choice. The strength or degree of the commitment of an individual is dependent upon the amount of belief or faith he has in the choice he made to produce a result he values. For example, a person chooses and commits himself to a political philosophy because he thinks that particular political philosophy will result in the best government; a leader chooses a type of leadership because he believes that type of leadership will result in the best patient care. *Choice* is one of the key activities of commitment. Agencies with policies on personnel evaluation that have been previously established by either the administration or by employees do not offer a choice between "to evaluate" or "not to evaluate." However, within every situation is some element of choice. The choices may be about how evaluations shall be done, who will participate, or the procedure to be used. Within the prescribed policy restrictions, personnel choices made in the full knowledge of limits of choice and alternatives available give the individual or group the beginnings of commitment. Commitment grows through seeing the choices implemented and feeling that the outcome of evaluation will be worthwhile.

PREDICTIVE PRINCIPLE: *Involvement of personnel in all phases of the evaluatory process increases belief in the fairness and accuracy of the evaluation, establishes a commitment to the evaluation, and increases motivation to utilize the results.*

Within agency structure each employee cannot be involved in every phase of the evaluation process. Employers usually classify personnel positions based upon administrative organization and defined patient and fiscal policies. Job descriptions are usually initially drafted by administrative personnel, but as an agency matures, professional performance committees may be created to represent employees in the activities of writing or revising job descriptions, establishing standards of practice, and developing criteria to determine if those standards have been met. Involvement of personnel who are to be affected by the committee's endeavors at all levels of evaluation will give the committee a wider base of support and will enable the committee to receive the necessary feedback to make valid decisions.

Employees can be involved in the formalized process of evaluation through participation activities using prescribed agency tools. Informal ongoing evaluation is pervasive in all nursing activities whether recognized and labeled or not. Individuals or groups who identify the ongoing nature and use of evaluations, formal or informal, and who can establish self-expectations designed to meet needs will quickly establish commitment to evaluation. The effectiveness of evaluation in improving patient care will become strikingly clear in a short span of time.

STANDARDS OF PRACTICE AND CRITERIA OF EVALUATION

Nursing organizations have become increasingly active in the area of establishing standards of professional performance. The most obvious milestone in setting minimum standards of practice was the instigation of the licensure examination, a measure for allowing an individual to practice nursing in a given state. Currently, most agencies have committees composed of representatives of the working group that establishes standards of practice and exercises control over the quality of nursing care in an agency. Standards of practice for all levels of nursing service personnel and the criteria necessary to measure behavior by those standards are the subject of this section.

Criterion, taken from the Greek word *kriterion*, is a means for judging. A criterion is a standard for measuring or a test by which something can be judged or tried. Adequate and accurate criteria enable adequate and accurate evaluations.

Isobel Stewart first developed guidelines in 1919 by which a procedure could be effectively standardized. Since that time, these have been modified and adapted by nurses and hospital associations for use in evaluating procedures and personnel. Stewart's criteria are modified here and slightly expanded, but they remain basically as she developed them. These criteria may be applied to any nursing activity and can be useful as guides to develop standards of practice and criteria of evaluation for the measurement of quality. *Stewart's criteria (modified)* * are as follows:
1. Safe and comfortable for the patient, nurse, and others
2. Technologically and therapeutically as advanced care as modern technology and science permits

---

*Stewart, I. M.: Possibilities of standardization in nursing techniques, Mod. Hosp., June, 1919.

3. Efficient and economical in time, energy, and supplies (the degree and priority of economy of time, energy, and supplies are legislated by the demands of criteria 1 and 2)

The three key words, "safe," "advanced," and "efficient," must be defined meaningfully for practical everyday use in evaluation. Each evaluating group may wish to discuss and define these words to their own satisfaction. A brief definition for each is suggested below:

1. Safe—will not harm the client or nurse physically or emotionally. Does not violate the client's physiologic, emotional, religious, or cultural integrity. Safety implies that the nurse will choose among available alternative actions. These actions will have the greatest potential for accomplishing the desired goal with the least risk of an undesirable consequence.
2. Advanced—use of skills and equipment and making decisions or exercising judgment based upon the latest available knowledge in physical, biologic, behavioral, and social sciences.
3. Efficient—the greatest amount of results with the least waste. Efficient does not mean merely "fast." It means effective, productive, and adequately fulfilling a purpose with the best possible use of the energy, time, and materials available.

PREDICTIVE PRINCIPLE: *Clear and concise role delineation and job descriptions enable employee, employer, and client to know the duties and responsibilities of the job.*

Role delineation and job descriptions are discussed in Chapter 4 and will not be repeated here.

Employees need copies of job descriptions available to them for all job classifications. Job descriptions help all employees to know what every other employee was hired to do. It is equally important for a care giver to know what his job is *not* as well as to know what it *is*. Nursing roles and job descriptions, clearly described in terms of relevance of each item to nursing practice, provide an objective way to ascertain if goals have been reached. If the job description is vague or if it ends with "and such other duties as may be required," the employee will not know what direction to take or what goals and objectives will be considered as most significant when outcomes are surveyed. Vague criteria in setting up job descriptions lead to a guessing game. Participants need to know areas of overlapping responsibility and areas of differing responsibility. Clear job descriptions are the nucleus of all subsequent evaluative activities.

PREDICTIVE PRINCIPLE: *Standards of performance and clear criteria for measuring performance increase the objectivity and validity of evaluation.*

The difference between performance standards and criteria of evaluation can be unclear. *Standards of performance* are usually general minimal standards established to govern the quality of nursing care. These standards definitively describe safety and expertise necessary for acceptable performance of the job. *Criteria of evaluation* enable the evaluator (care giver, client, nurse-leader, supervisor, or worker) to determine the *degree* and *extent* to which the evaluatee is performing in relationship to the established minimal standard.

Objectivity and validity in evaluation of performance are ideals that are never completely attained. *Objectivity* means unprejudiced, based upon real evidence, and uninvolved with self or at least minimally influenced by subjective involvement. Objectivity, though not completely attainable, can be controlled to some extent through the use of criteria as guides for making judgments and by remaining sensitive to and aware of biases and feelings.

Validity is the degree and extent to which the evaluation tool measures what it was intended to measure. Validity has two basic elements: (1) *reliability,* the degree and extent that an evaluation measures something, and (2) *relevance,* the degree and extent that it actually does measure what it is intended to measure. A criterion can measure reliably without measuring relevantly, and vice versa. However, a criterion must be both reliable and relevant for it to be valid.

The following is an example in which job classification, qualifications, standards of practice, and criteria of evaluation are followed through for one area of responsibility.

The Cedar Valley Visiting Nurse Association employs several levels of personnel who give nursing care on a team basis. LVNs are employed to perform specified functions. The following information is taken from performance materials provided to all personnel. One small area has been chosen to simplify the process. These items are not to be construed as complete.

Job classification:	Licensed vocational nurse.
Job qualifications:	Licensure by the state and one year of hospital or nursing home experience.
Other requirements:	Two character references; two professional performance references; and two formal interviews with designees of the Visiting Nurse Association.
Job description:	Will, under the supervision of a Registered Nurse, give basic care to designated patients. This includes appropriate hygienic care; special mouth, pubic, and foot care; oral medications and specified treatments.
Standards of practice:	Will exercise safety in the care of patients and will seek assistance or guidance when needed. Will collaborate with the team leader in making decisions about procedure.
	Hygienic care is expected to be performed to the following standards: Mouth: Mucosa and teeth clean, breath fresh.
Criteria of evaluation:	Mouth care: Gives routine mouth care to appropriate patients. Observes when other than routine mouth care is needed.
	Administers special mouth care procedures when necessary.
	Uses equipment appropriate to the type of mouth care to be given.
	Exercises safety precautions to protect the patient from injury (aspiration, gum or buccal abrasions).
	Protects self from contamination or contagion.
	Uses procedure requiring minimum expenditure of effort for both patient and nurse with maximum amount of comfort for both.
	Follows latest and most up-to-date directives about procedure.
	Displays economic use of time and equipment (for both agency and patient).

Use of a tool similar to the above for all nursing activities will provide participants with evaluative structure. (Note that the criteria for evaluations spelled out in behavioral terms facilitate the assessment process.)

Structure provides a measure of safety for both evaluator and evaluatee by making objectivity more achievable. A nurse-leader can have positive or negative feelings about the LVN but if the procedure has been performed and the criteria met as written, then personal feelings are less likely to influence evaluative judgment.

The *standard of performance* "mucosa and teeth clean, breath fresh" could be labeled a "relevant criterion." If an evaluator looked at the mouth of the patient and it exhibited clean mucosa and teeth and the patient's breath was odorless, the evaluator could unequivocally state that the standard had been achieved. The clean mouth indicates only that the desired result has been attained. Accurate evaluation of the practice used to accomplish the standard must be obtained by other means. The *list of criteria* is both relevant and reliable if, when used, the criteria measure the fact that a clean mouth was achieved (the criteria are relevant) and that the procedure was done with the appropriate equipment, the use of safety precautions, the least amount of effort, the latest technology, and the greatest economy (therefore the criteria are reliable).

Standards of performance and clear criteria for measuring performance provide both the evaluator and the evaluatee with guidelines for what constitutes good patient care. With these guidelines, value judgments can be made, and criteria of evaluation can unequivocally establish specific behavior expectations for excellence of nursing care.

PREDICTIVE PRINCIPLE: *Evaluation of individual and small group activity necessitates establishment of criteria for the evaluation process.*

Nurse practitioners who function independently or in small groups are answerable for both the tangibles and the intangibles of nursing and are expected to engage in a broad spectrum of roles, demonstrating the degree of expertise inherent in each of the roles.

The criteria used to evaluate the profession at large can be applied to individual or group practice. Following are some pivotal questions posed for making evaluative judgments:

1. Is the care giver or group leader legally qualified for the role?
2. Does authority for individual or group action lie with the participants, and if group effort is in process, is there an interdependent relationship?
3. Is there provision for individuals to pursue independent practice and to utilize one another as resource persons?
4. Are goals designed to meet the needs of the client or patient and practitioner?
5. Do care givers have a part in the development of goals, and are they committed to their fulfillment?
6. Are policies and job descriptions available that explain what is expected of each member, and are the members cognizant of their meaning, and are the expectations fulfilled?
7. Are nursing care plans formulated and implemented?
8. Does the care giver receive self-improvement and professional development through a well-designed educational program?
9. Do nurse members manifest behaviors indicating attitudes of satisfaction with their roles?

10. Is there evidence of nondiscriminatory behavior?
11. Is there a systematic design for evaluation of personnel and nursing care with respect to themselves and the total organization?

PREDICTIVE PRINCIPLE: *A contract meeting enables the accountable nurse and the client to determine whether the contract has been met.*

Nurses who are directly accountable to their patients and families, such as in the practice of primary care, bear responsibility for their services. Agreements for nursing care may be entered into between the patient and nurse, the health agency and the care giver, or the physician and the nurse. Implicit in the concept of accountability is obligation, liability, and trustworthiness. At the onset of employment a client and/or his family confers with the nurse for the purpose of mutual assessment, sharing of philosophy and expectations, and a review of policies and procedures held by the employing person or agency. This is the time for the care giver and client to negotiate and to make the decision to accept or reject the conditions as they are delineated. Inherent in the agreement is reciprocal accountability to see that provision for on-going processes for alteration of plans and evaluation as necessary for meeting expectations are implemented.

The nurse-practitioner will (1) determine and accept responsibility for leadership role, (2) identify his own and the client's capabilities and limitations, (3) set realistic scope and limitations of performance for self and client, (4) promote a climate for collaborative and cooperative communication, (5) make self available to patients, families, and other interested members of the health team for reporting, (6) develop problem-oriented care plans with the client and/or family, (7) carry prescribed plan into action and receive feedback from client and others about the results of the service, (8) seek assistance from appropriate resources when necessary, and (9) evaluate quality of performance and initiate steps for necessary changes or modification.

PREDICTIVE PRINCIPLE: *Use of appropriate assessment tools and sufficient evaluative data gathered from varied situations increase the validity of the conclusions.*

Nursing practice is validated through informal and formal means. No single style has been found to be consistently superior to another. Most individuals and health agencies utilize more than one technique, depending on (1) the purpose of the evaluation, (2) the availability of resources, and (3) the expertise and preference of those involved in the appraisal process.

Evaluation process takes the form of *informal* and *formal evaluation*. *Informal evaluation* may consist of (1) observation of an individual's work performance while he is engaged in nursing functions, (2) on the job, incidental face-to-face work and/or collaboration, (3) reflections offered during a meeting or conference, (4) reactions of an involved person, such as a patient, family member, or staff person, or (5) noting the effects of a worker's actions on patients, families, personnel, or environment. *Formal assessment* includes many methods. Nurses most often utilize (1) anecdotal recordings, (2) checklists based upon preestablished criteria, (3) dialogue based on one-to-one and group exchange,

(4) rating scales, and (5) cumulative records of activities engaged in for professional growth and/or advancement. Nurses may avail themselves of other methods, such as written and computer tests and other technologic testing devices. Practitioners can test their evaluative skills individually and collectively by viewing a filmed or taped nursing action and then assessing the situation. Videotaping with instant replay is a most appropriate device for the assessment of some nursing activities. Microtelevision can be used in actual or simulated settings. Evaluation of verbal and nonverbal interaction is particularly subject to this method.

All these avenues are most effective when there is commitment to the evaluation process by the evaluator, the person being evaluated, and the receiver of the information.

Anecdotal recording. An anecdote is a brief account of an incident and is an important means of illuminating evidence for evaluation. The anecdotal note has both advantages and disadvantages. The device is useful for frequent observations of short durations where variations in situations and personalities preclude advance determination of behavior. With this mechanism, it is possible to discover trends of conditions and behavior over a period of time. In many ways the anecdotal notes are superior to check lists or rating scales because observers are not forced into rigid structure in describing behavior. However, it is the very latitude of anecdotal notes that often leads to difficulty. The tool also provides a means for recording a description of a specific situation that could not have been anticipated and to tell how the individual acted in said situation. The anecdotal note is a means for describing a nurse's experience with a person or group. The anecdotal method is useful for recording and evaluating patient progress. Essentially, nurses' notes are one form of anecdotal record since they outline serially factual information with definite reference to the patient's progress. Other uses for this mode include validating technical skills, dialogue, and interpersonal relationships.

In any of these areas the behavioral pattern may vary from person to person and situation to situation. Although the general conditions and behaviors can be prescribed beforehand, the specific activities will be determined by circumstances incident to the occasion.

For maximum clarity, an anecdotal notation should include (1) a description of the particular occasion, (2) a delineation of the behavior noted, indicating who, what, why, when, where, and how, and (3) the evaluator's opinion or estimate of the incident and/or behavior. Decisions concerning what to observe and record are made on the basis of previously determined criteria, formal and informal. For expediency, the evaluator will develop a code or an abbreviated system for recording to facilitate speedy and accurate memorandums.

Perhaps the greatest difficulty in the use of anecdotal notes is the matter of developing some relationships among the various notations. Before it is possible to get impressions of the overall behavior in a given period of time, it is necessary to organize the descriptive notes. Often the notes bear little or no relationship to one another, and for this reason it is difficult to use them. The burden of organizing the notes falls on the observer or on the person who is attempting to interpret the meaning of the notes in relation to the evaluatee's behaviors.

Checklist. By definition, a checklist is a grouping of items by which something may be confirmed or verified. The checklist could be called a behavioral inventory. The checking process implies that standards and criteria are available for gauging items. The inspection procedure requires scrutiny of behavior under investigation. Checklists are most useful for determining the status of tangible items, such as inventory and maintenance of equipment and supplies. They have the advantage that items to be observed can be determined in advance and will be the same criteria used in each situation. Checklists are of some use as yardsticks for appraisal of nursing skills and techniques. There is no guarantee, however, that the observed behavior is a persistent one and that the procedure will provide a representative picture of the individual under surveillance.

Checklists applied in nursing attempt to itemize behaviors that are considered important elements of a task. One approach is to list satisfactory behaviors in a column; then determine the worker's overall performance on the basis of the items. For example, in observing administration of medications, the evaluator looks to see if the evaluatee: (1) checks physician's orders against nursing medication cards, (2) prepares the medication accurately using prescribed procedure, (3) identifies the patient and checks the medication card against the patient's wristband, (4) administers the medication, and (5) accurately charts medication given. It is recommended that only significant behaviors essential for a successful performance be included on the checklist. Only those behaviors that, if omitted or performed incorrectly, would make the difference between successful performance and unsuccessful performance should be included. The checklist does not lend itself well to evaluating patient progress, dialogue, or interpersonal relationships.

Rating scale. The rating scale, quite similar to the checklist, is another type of evaluation tool used in describing observed skills and performance. The basis of the rating device consists of such items as descriptive paragraphs, sentences, or phrases to serve as guidelines for the evaluator. Unlike the checklist, the rating scale may involve judgments as to quantitative and qualitative abilities. Such rating scales at the lower end might range from "incapable of performing a given task" to "poor" or "unsatisfactory." The scale will at its higher limits use such descriptive terms as "excellent," "outstanding," or "exceptional."

Some scales for the rating of performance employ the numerical system, using "one" to indicate the lowest behavioral pattern and "ten" or more to indicate the highest. The evaluator may fabricate a scale according to his own design and check behavioral patterns as occurring "consistently," "frequently," "sometimes," or "never." These numbers or words are ill defined, and only the evaluator may know what the evaluatee's level of performance and achievement is.

The rating scale is usually reserved for formal evaluation procedures, such as assessment of an employee or evaluatee at the end of a designated period, and is frequently associated with retention, promotion, and tenure. The device is comparative in nature. The rating is based on retrospective recordings and observations and is subject to human errors associated with recall and interpretation. This tool is most useful when each unit on the rating scale is identified and listed in terms of specific behaviors or circumstances.

A well-calibrated rating scale will consider (1) individual preparation for the role, (2) work setting and environment, (3) functions in relation to agency criteria, and (4) interpersonal relationships. Maximal utilization of the assessment tool depends upon involved individuals having prior knowledge of, participation in, acceptance of, and commitment to the content and use of the rating scale.

PREDICTIVE PRINCIPLE: *Use of the self-evaluation process promotes growth and development of the appraisor and contributes to better quality of care.*

Self-evaluation is used by everyone from childhood to senescence. The ability to be critical in assessing one's own performance is a mark of maturity and an integral part of nursing practice. Self-evaluation is implicit and continuous in the nursing process at every level of care giving. Self-evaluation has many valuable effects. The one engaged in introspection seeks to (1) obtain estimates of his level of achievement, (2) acquire meaningful information to assist with improvement in nursing practice, (3) gain information for self-improvement, growth and development, and the achievement of personal goals in a socially acceptable manner, and (4) enhance and improve human relations.

Self-rating can be heavily influenced by the individual's tendencies to overestimate or underestimate his own capabilities or achievements. Much success of self-evaluation programs depends upon the preliminary preparation of the participants to recognize their own strengths and weaknesses and to be as objective as possible in rating personal performance. Provided with adequate and procedural criteria for the assessment process and with various other appropriate tools, the individual can evaluate his progress in relation to these objectives, subject to constant reexamination and feedback. Self-evaluation is connected with personal goals, self-perception, self-confidence, and feelings of competence or incompetence. Most people have a fairly accurate picture of themselves and their abilities, but communication of self-evaluation is overlaid with many factors. Some of these are (1) who is reading the evaluation, (2) how the evaluation will be used, (3) the social acceptability of the self-judgment, and (4) peer pressures. If the care giver's self-appraisal threatens a job, promotion, salary increase, prestige or peer regard, it is unlikely that the assessment will be articulated and communicated, If, as is often the case, social pressure decries extremely high self appraisals, and the individual values social appraisal, the care giver's self evaluation is not likely to reflect areas of high competence. If (1) the evaluation is geared to citing goals for self, degrees to which goals have been realized, and plans for goal attainment, (2) the self-evaluation is to be used as a record of and provision for growth, and not as a means for punishment or reward, and (3) the self-evaluation report is confidential within preestablished limits and constraints, then self-evaluation is an accurate and useful tool and is likely to be effective when used in conjunction with other devices.

PREDICTIVE PRINCIPLE: *Participation of patient or client in the evaluation of care contributes to an accurate and composite assessment.*

As the recipient of care, the patient or client is in a strategic position to become involved in the verification of the effectiveness of his care. Basic to this concept is the belief that (1) care givers and recipients will have a vested interest in outcomes, (2) they will want to assume reciprocal responsibility for the implementation and revision of plans for care administered, (3) plans and evaluations will have a greater depth and increased objectivity when more than one person is involved, and (4) participation in the development and assessment of his care expedites and individualizes the patient's treatment and well-being.

Some clients are unable or simply do not wish to participate in planning for their health needs. This factor does not negate the feasibility of client contribution to the collection of evaluative data. The nurse observes the client's behavior and verbalizes subjective data. If the patient demonstrates that the objectives have been fulfilled, the desired evidence is acquired.

One approach to client evaluation is to establish the process on a continuum basis and to develop collaboratively with him a care plan that considers all phases of the process—assessment, problem identification, formulation of plans for nursing action, and planning for evaluation and implementation.* Nursing prescriptions are prepared with the client or patient and his family, and with the help of other members of the health team if needed. A copy is left with the patient. Updating and changing the care program is continuous and is done in conjunction with the client. This participatory mechanism provides an uncomplicated system for client evaluation. It is simple to assess the quality of various aspects of patient care, taking into consideration his knowledge of the treatment and the realization that it has been completed.

A checklist or questionnaire is another means of obtaining client data. Information gleaned from these tools usually refers to care already given (for example, "Did you feel nursing service was adequate?" "What more would you have liked to the nurse to do?" "Were your medications and treatments administered according to plan?" "Were you taught how to use the exchange plan in preparing your meals?" "Can you use the exchange plan now that you are home?"). These serve as input for assessing nursing action in general. The questionnaire or checklist designed to determine the discharged patient's understanding of his home care plan elicits information that assists the primary nurse in maintaining a continuous and comprehensive follow-up.

Although the client is encouraged to contribute ideas and approaches to problem-oriented treatment, the responsibility for developing, maintaining, implementing, and evaluating care rests with a particular nurse, who is held accountable for this service.

PREDICTIVE PRINCIPLE: *A limited number of observations on an incidental basis jeopardizes the accuracy of evaluations.*

PREDICTIVE PRINCIPLE: *Informal and formal assessments that are noted and recorded systematically provide significant input to the evaluation process.*

Observations of completed tasks can give an unreliable picture of performance. For example, the nurse-leader walks into a patient's room one hour after the change of the morning shift and finds the patient clean, neatly groomed, bed

---

*Bower, F. L.: The process of planning nursing care: a theoretical model, St. Louis, 1972, The C. V. Mosby Co., chap. 1.

freshly made, and the unit straight and uncluttered. Without additional data the nurse-leader could conclude that the nurse assigned to this patient was efficient and thorough. More complete data might reveal (1) that this patient was first on the list and therefore was cared for first regardless of the fact that another patient wanted early care so that she would be ready for a long-awaited visit from a loved one; (2) that the patient's receiving such efficient and thorough care was at the expense of the patient's breakfast, which became cold while waiting for the care giver to complete the care; (3) that the linen was piled upon the floor while the bed was being changed; or (4) that the patient was bathed in one small pan of water, which was not changed during the bath.

Value judgments made on one performance, the end product of a performance without reference to the process, or on many performances in the same situation can be erroneous because of lack of a variety of observations that would validate or refute previous judgments. For instance, a practitioner may use aseptic technique smoothly, correctly, and consistently when emptying catheter bags but may contaminate unknowingly when changing a sterile dressing. The criterion, "practices sterile technique with a high degree of skill," may be true when the nurse is performing one task and not true when performing another.

Both informal and formal input become significant if noted systematically and recorded as consistently as possible. The evaluation process is a means of determining the professional characteristics of an individual or a group. Similar behaviors as recorded in the evaluator's notes or tabulations indicate that a set of actions is predominately exhibited. Desirable behaviors that are rarely manifested are not given high priority when assessments are made; however, isolated achievements might become significant when motivation and potential are discussed.

Undesirable behaviors are important to consider. Again, isolated incidences are not used as conclusive data unless they become significant to the safety or welfare of the client. The right to be "human," or to improve, includes provision for making some mistakes without penalty or guilt. The evaluator's primary responsibility is to observe and note those behaviors exhibited most frequently and to deal with them. The aggregate of these samples gives a more reliable basis for determining a trend of behavior.

PREDICTIVE PRINCIPLE: *Valid interpretation of data depends upon equitable evaluation of input.*

Information gleaned from evaluation procedures may be meaningful only if they are used constructively and interpreted correctly. Judgments about the assignment of relative weight or value of each factor under consideration often become the responsibility of the nurse-leader, who will follow prescribed guidelines*: (1) client and nurse safety, (2) advanced knowledge and technology, (3) client comfort, (4) efficient use of time, and (5) cost effectiveness.

Other factors of an equitable evaluation of input for consideration are as follows:

---

*Stewart, I. M.: Possibilities of standardization in nursing techniques, Mod. Hosp., June, 1919.

1. Objective assessments should receive greater weight than subjective judgments.
2. When one person is evaluated and more than one individual is involved, the evaluators' impressions of the incident are diluted because it is difficult to determine the extent of each member's participation and the qualitative assistance obtained from extraneous sources.
3. Time is a factor in calibrating certain skills.
4. No single methodology should constitute the basis for success or failure in any nursing effort.

PREDICTIVE PRINCIPLE: *The evaluator who establishes mutual trust and confidence with the evaluatee and who is familiar with the criteria of evaluation increases the accuracy and usefulness of the evaluation.*

When the evaluator and evaluatee have a trusting relationship, the anxiety about evaluation is somewhat reduced. The extent to which evaluation activities cause anxiety, however, is directly related to what the person being evaluated stands to gain or lose. Evaluation that is constant and ongoing, and has as its objective the improvement of patient care through the upgrading of performance, becomes so much a part of routine and everyday nursing relationships that threat is reduced. On the other hand, the care giver who is in danger of being removed from the job, being suspended or relieved of responsibilities, or demoted *is* threatened. It is unrealistic to expect that the person or persons responsible for evaluating this person will be able to establish a relationship that is free of all anxiety.

Evaluations which result from cooperative effort and are accompanied by qualitative explanations that elucidate conclusions enable behavioral changes to be effectuated. Job descriptions, standards of practice, and criteria of evaluations all contribute to the ability to participate in evaluations. An employee who knows what constitutes a "good" or "bad" activity can recognize his own success or failure and take the initiative in corrective action. Consistently accurate self-evaluation is the ultimate achievement of evaluative activities, for it enables self-perpetuating growth.

The effect of evaluative comments on member behavior is related to the manner and intent of the message. Positive comments such as "You did a very good job on that," or "That was a fine bit of work you just did," serve to boost the morale of the worker and encourage continued high-level performance. Negative remarks create varied feelings ranging from the desire to improve to deep hostility toward the evaluator without a change in the undesirable behavior. Negative comments are very likely to be accompanied by an explanation of the reason for the criticism, while positive comments are seldom accompanied by explanation. It is important for the evaluatee to have information about *why* a behavior is "good" or "bad" so that the characteristics of the behavior can be either identified and repeated or changed.

Whether the evaluation is informal or formal, the evaluator bears in mind the need to preserve the integrity of the person or group being evaluated. Positive feedback, earned and given appropriately, contributes to the morale of each individual involved in the evaluation procedure.

Negative feedback also is essential for growth, as is positive feedback, and although it is often more difficult to give and to receive, it provides essential data. Withholding feedback of any kind, positive or negative, is an ultimately hostile act because it robs another person of data he needs to make intelligent choices and behavioral changes.

PREDICTIVE PRINCIPLE: *The degree to which the value systems of the evaluator and the evaluatee coincide influences their interpersonal relationships and directly affects the evaluation process.*

The dynamics of personal interaction and decisions are not wholly shaped by policies, job descriptions, and agreements. The conditions under which an individual operates and his perception of himself and others are the result of his value system. Value systems affect attitudes, which permeate and influence all contacts and have a direct effect on the task of evaluation. The bulk of administrative science literature in recent years emphasizes interpersonal relationships and the manner in which informal relations affected by values enhance or subvert interaction and organizational structure.

Interpersonal relationships are broad in scope, complex in nature, and constantly shifting. An attitudinal survey is a helpful part of the evaluation procedure. A cluster of attitudes recorded over a period of time assists the nurse-leader in guiding members toward positive directional goals. When guidelines are vague, evaluators may rely upon discriminatory behaviors and may tend to introduce ascriptive criteria, such as race, religion, sex, age, social background, personal connections, and friendships (Chapter 1).

A recent study of a major industrial firm supported the need for a well-defined and clearly understood policy to avoid discriminatory reaction. It was concluded that interpersonal pressures have their greatest impact upon a manager's decisions when he is not fully aware of policy; also, the manager's personality and values have their greatest impact upon his decisions when he is not certain of procedural format.* Assessments become ability oriented when objective criteria for the administration of patient care is considered, and knowledge, creativity, and job performance take precedence. Values are a part of each person and therefore influence evaluation. Clarity about's one's own standards and those of the evaluatee help keep value systems in perspective.

DISPOSITIONAL ACTIVITIES

Dispositional activities are those functions that channel the evaluative information to the appropriate source. Not all evaluation activities are such that a formal disposition is required.

Most evaluative feedback is verbal or behavioral and occurs between the evaluator and the evaluatee. This type of evaluation is incidental and frequent throughout a working day; it is seldom translated into a formal report. Behaviors, such as a frown from a co-nurse when a requested diabetic urine is obtained

---

*Quinn, R. P., Tabor, J. M., and Gordon, L. K.: The decision to discriminate: a study of executive selection, Ann Arbor, Mich., 1968, Institute for social research, The University of Michigan Press.

late or a smile when the diabetic urine results are obtained on time, are evaluative in nature and act as reinforcers of desired behaviors.

Evaluations that are more formal, but still not written or reported, take place in the form of conferences. Unwritten and informal evaluations not reported to others should be based on the same criteria used for written reports. The evaluator has some purpose for scheduling such conferences, which necessitates pre-planning of procedures that will facilitate accomplishment of the goal. The form and timing of the formal evaluative information depends upon how the evaluation is to be used. Evaluative information may be dispensed to any person involved in primary care or independent nursing practice or in the line organization who has official access to the information or his designee. Among these may be any one or all of the following:

1. The client
2. The individual employee
3. The person evaluated
4. The head nurse
5. The supervisor
6. The nursing service personnel
7. Official committees of the agency
   a. Retention committee
   b. Professional standards committees
   c. Personnel promotion committees
   d. Research or data collection committees
8. Personnel office

The form the dispositional activity takes can be in any one or a combination of the following:

1. Verbal feedback
2. Behavioral feedback
3. Written memo
4. Formal evaluation using prescribed form
5. Signed official or personal letter

All evaluations, regardless of the form used, must be substantiated and qualified with first-hand evidence of the application of established criteria.

PREDICTIVE PRINCIPLE: *Frequent feedback on performance by a qualified evaluator, based on appropriate observations, reinforces desired behaviors and increases awareness of areas that need improvement.*

PREDICTIVE PRINCIPLE: *Negative evaluative feedback accompanied with suggestions for improvement helps the evaluatee to change his behavior to more acceptable levels of performance.*

Feedback is the most important factor influencing behavioral change. The most effective evaluative feedback is given at the time the incident occurs. The closer the feedback occurs to the time of the incident the more nearly the participants can place it in context and the more meaningful it will be.

Formal written evaluations given in response to agency policy or to a felt need should be based on agency job descriptions, standards of practice, and criteria of evaluation. If all these are not available, attempts can be made to acquire other evaluative tools. The American Nurses' Association, National League for Nursing, and American Hospital Association are reliable sources for assistance.

Effective evaluations are perpetrated *up* as well as *down* the administrative hierarchy. However, staff members seldom offer any but informal and incidental evaluations of agency superiors. The nature of threat and the opportunity for retaliation make evaluations of administrative superiors a high-risk situation.

PREDICTIVE PRINCIPLE: *An evaluation process that includes reciprocal participation both vertically and horizontally provides an avenue for high level morale and job satisfaction.*

Assumption of responsibility for one's actions and individual growth and development require feedback data. There is no way to equate the democratic process with secrecy. The individual or group in question should not only see the progress report but also should actually be involved in the assessment process. The evaluator can then validate actions as they occur and are later discussed and recorded. There may remain unresolved differences of opinion in appraisal after attempts at clarification. In a fair manner and with the right to appeal in due process, opportunity should be provided for opposing views to be heard and recorded. The group or person being reviewed may request a third party report in defense of stated opinion. The evaluator may also wish to elicit assistance from outside sources, such as an immediate supervisor, nurse-leader, or allied health personnel in gathering data and in preparing the report.

All written evaluations should be read and signed by the evaluatee in the presence of the evaluators, and any rebuttal or confirmation that the evaluatee wishes to enclose can then be attached and forwarded to the appropriate agency official or committee.

APPLICATION OF PREDICTIVE PRINCIPLES IN EVALUATION OF PERSONNEL

An LVN encounters the head nurse in the hall and says, "I wish you'd place Mrs. Mitchell (an aide) somewhere else. I can't stand to work with her another minute!" The nurse asks, "What is going on?" After clarification, the head nurse determines the LVN believes Mrs. Mitchell is "not doing her job."

PROBLEM	PRINCIPLES	PRESCRIPTION
To validate whether Mrs. Mitchell is performing job requirements.	Standards of performance and clear criteria for measuring performance increase the objectivity and validity of evaluation. Involvement of personnel in all phases of the evaluation process increases belief in the fairness and accuracy of the evaluation, establishes a commitment to the	Make preliminary observations and assessments based on standards of performance and criteria. Inform Mrs. Mitchell that she is going to be evaluated. Determine if Mrs. Mitchell has job descriptions, standards of prac-

PROBLEM	PREDICTIVE PRINCIPLES	PRESCRIPTION
Validation of performance—cont'd	evaluation, and increases motivation to utilize the results. Clear and concise job descriptions enable employee and employer to know the duties and responsibilities of the job.	tice, and criteria, and initiate cooperative activities of evaluation.
	Evaluative data gathered from a variety of situations in sufficient quantity increase the objectivity and validity of evaluation.	Collect behavioral notations about Mrs. Mitchell's work; Mrs. Mitchell's evaluation about herself; and evaluation of patients cared for by her (made at various times of the work period, observing for the use of safety precautions, comfort measures, and efficiency).
	Frequent feedback on performance by a qualified evaluator, based upon appropriate observations, reinforces desired behaviors and increases awareness of areas that need improvement. Negative evaluative feedback accompanied with suggestions for improvement helps the evaluatee to change his behavior to more acceptable levels of performance.	Set time aside to compare data, draw conclusions, and design ways to improve. Record evaluation and make appropriate disposition of the information.

BIBLIOGRAPHY

BOOKS

Alexander, E. L.: Nursing administration in the hospital care system, St. Louis, 1972, The C. V. Mosby Co.

Armstrong, R. J., et al.: The development and evaluation of behavioral objectives, Worthington, Ohio, 1970, Charles A. Jones Publishing Co.

Biehler, R. F.: Psychology applied to teaching, Boston, 1971, Houghton Mifflin Co.

Durbin, R. L., and Springall, W. H.: Organization and administration of health care: theory, practice, environment, St. Louis, 1969, The C. V. Mosby Co.

Flanders, N. A.: Analyzing teaching behavior, Reading, Mass., 1970, Addison-Wesley Publishing Co., Inc.

Gagné, R. M.: Perspectives of curriculum evaluation, Chicago, 1967, Rand McNally & Co.

Gavelock, R. G.: A guide to innovation in education, Ann Arbor, Mich., 1970, Center for research on utilization of scientific knowledge, Institute for social research, The University of Michigan Press.

Hough, J. B., and Duncan, J. K.: Teaching: description and analysis, Reading, Mass., 1970, Addison-Wesley Publishing Co., Inc.

Litwack, S. R., and Wykle, M.: Counseling, evaluation and student development in nursing education, Philadelphia, 1972, W. B. Saunders Co.

Mager, R. F., and Pipe, P.: Analyzing performance problems, Belmont, Calif., 1970, Fearon Publishers.

Schweer, J. E.: Creative teaching in clinical nursing, ed. 2, St. Louis, 1972, The C. V. Mosby Company.

Shaffer, S. M., Indorato, K. L., and Deneselya, J. A.: Teaching in schools of nursing, St. Louis, 1972, The C. V. Mosby Company.

Warren, R. L.: Studying your community, New York, 1965, The Free Press.

PERIODICALS

Aiken, L., and Aiken, J.: A systematic approach to the evaluation of interpersonal relationships, Am. J. Nurs. **70**(4):863-867, 1970.

Bare, C. E.: Behavioral changes through effective evaluation, J. Nurs. Educ. **6**(11):7-9, 1967.

Cantor, M.: Standard V: education for quality care, J. Nurs. Admin., pp. 48-54, Feb.-March, 1973.

Clissold, G. K., and Metz, E. A.: Evaluation—a tangible process, Nurs. Outlook **14**(3):41-45, 1966.

Cochran, T. C., and Ransen, P. J.: Developing an evaluation tool by group action, Am. J. Nurs. **62**(3):94-97, 1962.

De Tornyay, R.: Measuring problem-solving skills by means of the simulated clinical nursing problem test, J. Nurs. Educ. **7**(10):3-8, 1968.

Kirsch, A. I.: Planning for a sensible health care system, Nurs. Outlook **20**(10):640-647, 1972.

Long, K. R.: Consumer controlled nursing, Nurs. Outlook **17**(9):51-54, 1969.

Marram, G. D.: Patients' evaluation of their care: importance to the nurse, Nurs. Outlook **21**(5):322-324, 1973.

Moore, M. A.: Philosophy, purpose and objectives: why do we have them? J. Nurs. Admin., pp. 9-14, May-June, 1971.

N. L. N. Testing Services: Let's examine, an annotated bibliography on measurement and evaluation. Part II. Nurs. Outlook **16**(6):52-53, 1968.

Ortelt, J.: The development of a scale for rating clinical performance, J. Nurs. Educ. **5**(1):15-17, 1966.

Palmer, M. E.: Cumulative record of personal and professional growth, Nurs. Outlook **14** (6):39-41, 1967.

Pardee, G., Hoshaw, D., Huber, C., and Larson, B.: Patient care evaluation is every nurse's job, Am. J. Nurs. **71**(10):1958-1960, 1971.

Peterson, G. G.: Evaluating the assignments head nurses make, Am. J. Nurs. **73**(4):641-644, 1973.

Rosen, A., and Abraham, G. E.: Evaluation of a procedure for assessing the performance of staff nurses, Nurs. Res. **12**:78-82, Spring, 1963.

Slee, V. N.: How to know if you have quality control, Hosp. Prog. **53**(1):38-43, 1972.

Topf, M.: A behavioral checklist for estimating the development of communication skills, J. Nurs. Educ. **8**(11):29-34, 1969.

CHAPTER SIX

Predictive principles for changing

BASIC GROUND RULES

Using clear communications and ground rules facilitates the interpersonal exchanges necessary for planned changes to occur.

Consideration of each other's ideas and opinions and application of interpersonal communication predictive principles by change participants develops a growing trust in membership and group process and concomitantly facilitates increasing effectiveness of problem solving.

CONDITIONS NECESSARY TO CHANGING

Failure of a nursing care delivery system to meet the needs of its practitioners, clients, and/or employers ensures changes in or the death of the system.

The breakdown of effectiveness of standard procedures and traditional organization causes an increase in anxiety of the individual nursing care giver.

Experiencing high anxiety levels provides a need for change or adaptation, accompanied by an increase in individual and collective energy.

Need for change or adaptation stimulates personal fantasies of solutions or anticipation of the achievement of objectives.

Free exchange of ideas about goals and subgoals enables the establishment of specific and legitimate goals and collaboration for their achievement.

Explicit participation and support of the administration for changes ensures the changing group has the power and authority to implement plans for change.

Creating environmental and operational conditions that nurture the change process supports the potential success of the change effort.

Group commitment to the change process itself instead of specific changes enables continuing investigation, growth, and improvement.

BASIC ORGANIZATIONAL PATTERNS FOR CHANGING

Use of an organizational pattern for changing that utilizes a theoretical framework for guiding the logistics of human resources in a task-oriented system promotes effective and efficient use of energy toward attainment of the goal.

BASIC PLANNING STRATEGIES FOR CHANGING

An explicit and definitive task analysis supports the ability of the client system to have an overall view of the subgoals and tasks to accomplish these goals.

Formation and assignment of task groups according to the task, time limitations, and capabilities of the change participants enables each member to contribute optimally.

Organization of change participants around components of task analysis decreases "power" focus and increases goal orientation of work groups.

Feedback from an alter group during the planning phase increases the probability that the group product will meet the staff needs, fulfill the task charge, and be useful to the target system.

Generating several alternative solutions to a problem to achieve a goal enables the group to select an alternative most nearly in keeping with group needs.

Explicit rewards or recognition of individual or group achievement reinforces changing behaviors and promotes continuing efforts toward realization of goals.

Stability is a mirage, an illusion, a nirvana for which one yearns or dreams. Individuals move through life seeking stability as knights sought the mythical Holy Grail. But life consists of balancing forces that pull, tug, and push in powerful energy fields. Nurses often feel caught in these forces, tossed and helpless in their grasp. The feeling of loss of control is frightening, and the energy drain in simply attempting to cope is tremendous. The energy exerted toward controlling self and others is often wasted because the forces of life's changes buffet people like a volleyball floating upon a river. The resultant sense of powerlessness is a devastating feeling, and anger, aggression, frustration, and depression are high correlates of this powerlessness.

Control is the key. However, to affect, influence, and facilitate changes rather than be tossed hopelessly by them, one must focus the energy of control on the *forces causing change,* not the *people who are buffeted* or caught in the forces. This strange paradox can be likened again to the volleyball on the river. The force, speed, direction, and temperature of the water in the river directly influence the inflation pressure within the ball and the direction and rapidity with which it moves. If the change agent wishes to control the ball, his most reasonable approach is to control the flow of water in the river. Volleyballs do not lend themselves to having rudders, sails, or engines placed on them for control of movement; neither do people. Volleyballs can be tethered to a rope or string, but such control severely limits their movement and makes them single direction oriented. Real, free moving direction is exerted by controlling the forces that regulate the flow of water. This can be accomplished by removing or adding rocks and boulders, leveling the terrain, smoothing the river bed, rechanneling a curve or damming up tributaries and reducing the water volume, or even altering the water temperature (by adding a power plant). Similarly, energy directed toward identifying and isolating the forces causing change, examining the consequences of controlling each of these forces, wisely selecting which consequence is desirable, and manipulating the force field is energy that has a payoff in a directly controlled and effective change program.

The context of nursing and its influence on nursing change

Nursing is a process or, if you prefer, a system and is subject to influences of other processes. Alterations in other processes or systems act as stimuli to nursing, and nursing responds to them either adaptively or maladaptively. The system that does not respond will not remain viable. The system that responds maladaptively may cease to be functional and thus becomes outmoded or unused. Nursing is an open system and is linked with other living processes. Nursing is influenced by and is responsive to stresses from such other operant systems as the political system, the social system, and the technologic system.

1. *The political system.* Funding patterns, such legislated matters as national health insurance, licensure and accreditation laws, nurse and other health worker practice acts, and educational legislation affecting nursing care delivery, client receipt, and nursing manpower production and distribution serve to constitute the political arena. This arena is the basic battleground for nursing care quality control, education and development, and delivery system

funding. Nursing leaders need to address themselves to the politics of health care and the subsequent cash flow patterns, which are derived from legislation on the community, state, and federal levels.

2. *The social system.* The characteristics of populations in social systems and their needs change. For instance, the values in the United States have shifted from the melting pot dream of complete amalgamation of ethnic and racial population to pridefully organized groups, with emphasis on cultural, racial, and ethnic uniqueness. The need system shifted when the value system changed. Population characteristics are constantly changing both nationally and in the specific environment of any nursing care group. The shift may be to concentrations of senior citizens in particular locations as retirement villages become popular. There may be high density areas for specific ethnic groups or for great numbers of young people as around colleges and universities. As mental hospitals empty and half-way houses, board and care homes, and other such group-living situations become more prevalent and preferred, concentrations of the disabled or socially maladapted will be more common. Other alterations are evidenced by changes in marriage patterns, the role of women, family dynamics, organizations and power groups, and trends in social values.

3. *The technologic system.* The technologic system affects nursing through various avenues. The equipment developed for health care giving and teaching makes nursing care pattern changes necessary. Transportation patterns are causing health care delivery modes to adapt. Mobile clinics, increasingly efficient urban transportation, satellite centers, and other nonhospital-oriented care systems are directly the effects of increased transportation technology. *Computer technology* perhaps offers the largest untapped potential for influencing modifications in nursing care. This potential is being implemented in some health care centers on trial bases with varying success. The near future will see computer banks utilized for central recording of patient information and for instant retrieval for solving nursing problems. The patient's chart will be a tape in a computer; his social security number will be the magic key to his cumulative health record, which will be easily transferred, with his permission, from one health arena to another, enabling the client's health care to become integrated. Nurses needing information relevant to the situation, from preoperative procedures to the order and sequence of diagnostic tests, may obtain this information with greatest efficiency by computerized instant data control.

Because of these and other forces, changes in nursing are gathering speed, and nurses are learning to respond to the needs for alteration, to control some of the variables influencing change, and thus to affect the direction, speed, and quality of innovations. In effect, the problem with modification is that change is not permanent; each ensuing experience brings another set of circumstances to be viewed, dealt with, and recycled into the change format.

Nurses cannot usually affect all the forces that make up the context of nursing and thereby influence nursing response to those forces. However, nurses can attain enough influence over the immediate variables affecting nursing care to govern the direction, rate, and expression of change in nursing. This chapter addresses itself to those areas over which nursing leaders can exercise influence and affect change.

The process of changing*

The process of changing is a process of both leadership and accountability. It is a method of organizational structure and management and a means of adaptation and problem solving. In the process of changing, the interdependent and mutually inclusive nature of all processes meaningful to nursing is obvious. Planned change is change with a purpose, devised to solve problems of nursing care through the use of behavioral science technologies. Planned change is a type of human engineering where theories of human behavior are applied so that intelligent choices and actions are made. *The process of changing deals with alterations by choice and deliberation and is distinctly different from change by indoctrination, coercion, natural growth, and accident. In all facets of nursing, appropriate application of behavioral science techniques can produce changes that are the result of collective and collaborative choice, that is, participatory changing.*

For any nursing care system to change and grow, practitioners must respond through participation and collaboration to the vast number of variables in the health needs system with constructive deliberate changes in ways and means of coping with health problems. The use of theories of change in all nursing care systems—individual client, family group, and community—is necessary to the creative element of nursing processes.

One of the most difficult problems facing change agents is the lack of a conclusive theory on how to implement changes. Many studies have been done on the mechanics, the dynamics of change. But according to Bennis,† there is no theory of changing. However, there are some propositions about effecting social change that can be used as guides for change in nursing.

Change theorists commonly refer to the components of the change process as follows:

Agent: Facilitator, social scientist, nurse (trained in the science of change)
Rate: Speed at which change takes place (evolutionary, slow, revolutionary, galloping)
Arena: Organization, institution (the place in which the change occurs, the environment of change)
Person: Target of change (client of change, the client system; may be an individual or a group)

The bureaucratic ways in which nursing care agencies are organized—the use of authoritative patterns of organization, the use of committee structure, and the use of parliamentary law for decision making—lock nursing care systems into stable and sometimes inflexible patterns of unproductive behavior. These practices mitigate against optimal participation, generation of the most workable alternatives, and maximum use of all participants' talents in planning for changes.

Nursing agencies, like most institutions, are organized around the military model of authoritarian structure. Employees fit into a line organization that

---

*The remainder of this chapter is adapted from Bevis, E. O.: Curriculum building in nursing: a process, St. Louis, 1973, The C. V. Mosby Co., chapters 4 and 8.

†Bennis, W. G.: Changing organizations, New York, 1966, McGraw-Hill Book Co., pp. 81-94 and 99-108.

stacks in groups or units toward people with more and more power and authority.

All authoritarian organizations use some modification of this military pattern. There are many variations of format, but basically each person is responsible, at least in name, for all that occurs beneath his level in the hierarchical setup. In this way, decisions are delayed while they are passed up the line for someone with "more authority to make decisions" to act upon. When groups organized in the traditional bureaucratic or hierarchical form of organization deny that this authoritarian pattern exists, it places people in the administrative positions of having to maintain the responsibility because of institutional organization but of having little or no authority because of the nursing group organization. Attempting to change the system can absorb energy that would be better used in making changes in nursing care giving and can effectively delay work to that end. Since the objective is usually nursing care improvement rather than institutional reorganization, a group can (for that objective) create a nursing organization that will facilitate work; for example, the staff can agree to try a different organizational mode for planning, creating, building, and testing change. Formal lines of operation can be maintained for other business and activities. The organizational problem is twofold: (1) how to get maximum participation by the total group involved with change and (2) how to make the changes flexible and responsive to society's or clients' needs. There are four categories of change factors that facilitate the two goals listed above: (1) basic ground rules, (2) conditions necessary to changing, (3) basic organizational patterns for changing, and (4) basic planning strategies for changing. "Basic" is used because the suggestions here are beginning ones; for each phase of change activities, the group may wish to modify, add to, alter, delete, or suspend some of the organizational modes, ground rules, or planning strategies, depending upon the needs of the moment.

BASIC GROUND RULES

During change, people become somewhat frightened of the future because it is an unknown. Change participants easily become suspicious that something is being put "over on them." People often feel isolated and powerless. Their usual power bases are dissolved, familiar landmarks disappear, and fear of having no influence over the changes often underlies some of the resistive behavior seen in groups. There are ways a change agent can avoid some of the difficulties resulting from the nebulosity of change. Ground rules for the group interaction involved in planning for and implementing changes can, when used consistently, help to decrease communication problems.

PREDICTIVE PRINCIPLE: *Using clear communications and ground rules facilitates the interpersonal exchanges necessary for planned changes to occur.*

Group work toward changing is facilitated if there are some basic operational ground rules for the accomplishment of objectives. Nurses working together for changes need to develop ground rules that facilitate change and promote healthy group relationships. It is possible to achieve both ends. Most often nursing staff working relationships have established patterns of interaction—some patterns that facilitate and some that inhibit functional communications. On any nursing staff, there are committees or groups that are powerful. Immediately upon the opening of an issue, pro and con groups draw their battle lines, and win-lose conflicts are generated. With people who have worked together for long periods of time, the "red flags" or "buttons" that will elicit known predictable reactions are familiar and assessable. Button pushing and red flag waving can be a favorite pastime or a smooth way to sidetrack an issue. There are no easy answers to the problem of establishing communication patterns that are more supportive, productive, and useful for facilitating change. An outside communication facilitator is invaluable to any group considering approaching change. Neutral, uninvolved facilitators can help group members look at transactions and interactions, analyze the communication factors, and establish more effective ways of communicating. The following list provides a sample of items groups might like to consider for operational ground rules. Each group will evolve its own list and supplement it as it is used. Following are some prescriptive interpersonal ground rules for change communications:

1. Try to have no surprises. Let everyone know in advance plans that are under way; peep previews, preliminary reports, and agreements to check out rumors will keep surprises at a minimum.

2. Provide as much informational input as possible. Part of the backbone of any planned change is the collection of data phase. "Hand outs," consultation with experts, training sessions, television, movies, and other audiovisual materials, circulation of helpful articles, and data discussion sessions prior to the time the information must be used help to provide the data base necessary to planned changes.

3. Make conflicts explicit and legitimate. Bring out hidden agenda items so that real issues can be handled. Legitimacy of conflict makes it possible to look for alternatives that meet every group's goals rather than locking into win-lose power struggles.

4. Identify high investment areas (areas of high feelings) and elicit the help of a neutral facilitator either from within the group or from a source unrelated to the problem or issue itself. This enables all factions to struggle or fight "fair," for a facilitator will ensure each participant's rights.

5. Make risks legitimate and failure salvageable and acceptable. Operating in small task areas or "bits and pieces" allows greater risks to be taken because if one small part fails, the whole system of changes is not likely to fall apart. Back-up systems are other alternatives for handling the problem if an original plan fails.

6. Make change in the middle of a trial run acceptable. Then if a plan being instituted is not working, alterations in the plan can be made without violating the group's preconceived notion that a trial run *has* to be run all the way through.

7. Try to make it necessary to analyze failure or the reasons a part of a program is not working so that alterations and changes are not precipitous

or without fair trial, or so that the parts of a plan that may be causing the problems can be changed.

8. Agree to respond to each other's contributions to the group—comments, needs, and behaviors. Acknowledgment of entering into the group process reinforces and encourages continuing contributions and provides feedback. To be unacknowledged or consistently erased leaves one having few behavioral cues, having a feeling of impotence and powerlessness, and feeling very alone in the group. Other participants are aware of nonresponsiveness and are reluctant to risk contributing and not being responded to. A simple agreement to say "amen" or use some "body language" that is an obvious acknowledgment is necessary to a developing sense of group power.

9. When complete win-lose deadlocks occur, agree to some form of action that will allow unlocking and saving of pride. Delay the issue or shuttle it to another time if necessary so that the group can be explicitly charged to look for alternatives that will meet criteria for a solution that pleases all. One way is to say, "What do we want in the solution that will fulfill the needs of both groups?" Then brainstorm for criteria. Try never to make a voting decision while in win-lose situations.

10. Delay making "final" decisions. Make tentative decisions, take a consensus, decide on a "trial" basis or accept something as a "provisional" or "working copy." Voting and recording in the minutes creates a feeling of finality that makes it more difficult for members of the change group to accept alterations. Minutes become "laws," and members refer to them to "win" battles. If records are needed, call them "notes on the conference on . . ." or "record of discussion."

PREDICTIVE PRINCIPLE: *Consideration of each other's ideas and opinions and application of interpersonal communication predictive principles by change participants develops a growing trust in membership and group process and concomitantly facilitates increasing effectiveness of problem solving.*

Free exchange of ideas is not possible without an atmosphere of trust. Trust is basic to the mechanisms of planned change and is developed through consistently respecting the rights and limits of others and in meeting the needs of the group and the individuals in the group. Continuing communication requires a set of changing, evolving, colleague-oriented, equally participative ground rules. In autocratic systems, loyalty is given to the institution or group, to the employer, "boss," or supervising personnel. Peer group relations are marked by competition and a win-lose attitude in the suggesting of goals or solutions.

In a group in which the safeguards of ground rules have been established, in which each group member assumes the responsibilities for the group's work and is accountable for the quality of the group's communications, several things occur:

1. Individual faith in the ability of the group to produce successfully increases.

2. Individual respect for members' ability to participate increases.

3. Trust in the group process increases.

4. Group skill in problem solving increases.
5. Win-lose discussions decrease as the group becomes increasingly skillful at designing a multiplicity of alternatives that are win-win.
6. Essential support for individuals becomes possible without sacrificing the goals of the group.
7. Loyalty to the profession of nursing and to colleagues begins to replace loyalty to agency or authority persons.

CONDITIONS NECESSARY TO CHANGING

The rapid changes occurring in society cause change "waves" that affect all facets of life. Rigid structures, like sea walls, take the brunt of change waves and crack under the constant battering. Flexibility enables people and institutions to survive battering by altered needs that make change inevitable.

PREDICTIVE PRINCIPLE: *Failure of a nursing care delivery system to meet the needs of its practitioners, clients, and/or employers ensures changes in or the death of the system.*

Change occurs when needs arise with which standard procedures and modes of behavior cannot cope. When new factors appear and many variables become part of a formally stable organization, new adaptive mechanisms are necessary to ensure continuity, quality, and efficiency of nursing care responses. Organizations, institutions, and individuals that have found a modus operandi that works for them tend to "fix" or "solidify" that operational system because the very fact that it works is reinforcing. Thus, when factors in the environment or some of the needs of consumers of the nursing care delivery system change, the system fails to respond by modifying its standard mode of operation, causing a decrease in efficiency, unmet needs, unachieved purposes, a decrease in quality care, and a reduction in nurse and employer satisfaction.

For instance, when the socially characteristic health needs or quality expectations of clients change, the nursing care delivery system may or may not respond to those changes. If the system does not alter with each new need or new variable, the changes begin to accrue and affect the relevancy of the whole care process. Eventually the variables—such as changes in the ethnic composition of the client group, shifting emphasis in the numbers of clients cared for at home rather than in the hospital, number of clients seeking nursing care, changing laws affecting nursing education and service, and greater participation of clients in their own health care—accrue. The system of nursing must either respond to those changes or remain rigidly unresponsive and therefore become increasingly irrelevant. Subsequently, the majority of the nurse's time is spent in coping with a series of crises generated by poor adaptation. Historically, nursing has had very few variables, for many factors were stable and dependable, and standard procedures and stylized care systems were the ways used to cope with those conditions. Now health care as a national concern is a focus of the energy of consumers, legislators, and health professionals. The variables are so many and the stable factors so few that standard, previously learned modes of operation will no longer serve. The cues in the nursing world that were formerly considered stable points of reference no longer exist. Nursing will either decline as a discipline or devise more flexible and versatile programs of service and education.

PREDICTIVE PRINCIPLE: *The breakdown of effectiveness of standard procedures and traditional organization causes an increase in anxiety of the individual nursing care giver.*

Anxiety is the signal of readiness to change. Even though mild anxiety is the natural state of an organism, a rise in the normal level of anxiety makes for discomfort, and nurses often seek to return to a more comfortable state of being. If change procedures are not instituted that will enable better coping with the new factors, anxiety will continue to increase until total efficiency is affected. Some nursing groups do not institute plans for changing until there are a limited number of alternatives, and change is then a matter of crisis. In this instance, change that is planned for long-term goals must be delayed while crisis intervention occurs, panic is controlled, or extreme anxiety states are lowered.

Crisis is a time when intense learning can occur, and rapid changes can be made. However, a change agent must be available during crisis to participate with the nursing group in crisis intervention activities. Changes are easier when nurses preplan and work out changes in advance. But when a care delivery crisis occurs because of legislation, administrative edict, client demands, or changes in the nursing care group composition, crisis can become the useful vehicle for changes.

PREDICTIVE PRINCIPLE: *Experiencing high anxiety levels provides a need for change or adaptation, accompanied by an increase in individual and collective energy.*

People in the anxiety need-to-change sequence exhibit greater work output. However, if there is no articulation of goals, the work output takes on the form of "busy work," of trying to make the obsolete system work successfully, of vicious circles, or of activities designed to control self and others. If the next phase of planned change is instituted, energy is available for work toward planning change. Nurses experiencing anxiety are open to alternatives and can learn new behaviors both for planning and for implementing changes. Change agents who can provide options, models, cues, stimulants, and otherwise facilitate solution-directed activities during anxiety help the group use their energy in positive ways. This phase of anxiety, when the energy output level is increased, is "prime time" for changing.

PREDICTIVE PRINCIPLE: *Need for change or adaptation stimulates personal fantasies of solutions or anticipation of the achievement of objectives.*

Everyone who is troubled dreams a dream of "trouble free." Fantasies occur, such as "if only this and that were so, all would be right with heaven and earth" and "if we had this or that in our agency, the millennium would be here." Everyone anticipates longingly the achievement of his private vision of how things could be better. One of the difficulties is that visions of improvement, visions of *how* things could be improved, and vision of "objectives" are *private*. As private objectives they have the connotation of illegitimacy, or being unacceptable. People fear offending other people—"power" people, vested interest groups, and friends. If the goals are shared at all, they are shared with a few chosen associates. When nurses share ideas and goals, they find others in the group have common dreams and goals. Aloneness is decreased, and objectives become legitimate.

PREDICTIVE PRINCIPLE: *Free exchange of ideas about goals and subgoals enables the establishment of specific and legitimate goals and collaboration for their achievement.*

Visions of the future can be translated into group objectives only if the group provides a time or a mechanism for articulation of ideas and fantasies about the future so that goals for work and criteria for changes can be established.

Change can be just a "happening," that is, a product of chance. Chance brings many alterations—some toward a desired end, some away from it. The ability to talk freely together as a group involved in changing promotes the realization of group goals through the mechanism of *making goals and means for reaching them legitimate, explicit topics for discussion.* Participation of those affected by changes at every level—administration, head nurses, staff nurses, LVNs, aides and students—generates a commitment to the change process itself and makes collaboration for specific tasks possible and desirable.

PREDICTIVE PRINCIPLE: *Explicit participation and support of the administration for changes ensures the changing group has the power and authority to implement plans for change.*

Every nursing organization has an administrator, a supervisor, a chief, a chairman, or a director. This person is, in the eyes of the institution, accountable to his superior for the activities of the staff, the delivery of care, and the success or failure of the developing change enterprise. Thus, no changes of major dimensions can occur without the consent and participation of the ranking persons. Because authority figures have and can exercise veto power or can influence administrators up the line to exercise veto power, the veto ability needs to be made explicit to the planning group. Inclusion of administrative persons in work (task groups, heuristics, findings) decreases surprise, keeps them involved with the changes being planned, and reduces the chance that vetoes will occur.

PREDICTIVE PRINCIPLE: *Creating environmental and operational conditions that nurture the change process supports the potential success of the change effort.*

For change to occur, certain conditions must be provided. The change agent seeks, in collaboration with others, to establish these conditions so that planned change can proceed. These conditions are as follows:

1. *Key organizational people must support and participate in the change.* In nursing care delivery system change, administrators, directors, committee chairmen, inservice education coordinators, physicians, and other key power people must support the idea of planned change as a total group effort. Since this means relinquishing some power to the group and exposing oneself in the group on a peer basis, it is, at first, a beginning acquiescence, but hopefully it

becomes a growing commitment. Dignified retirements, transfers, and resignations are not necessary except in rare instances. Trust, collaboration, peer relationships, and free exchange of ideas are *learned* phenomena, and with a skilled change agent, any group can learn these behaviors.

2. *The processes employed in change must be congruent with the philosophy, processes, and goals of change.* The ends do not justify the means, and the means employed for change must be of the same kind and caliber as the change that is desired. People learn as much from models as they learn from any other learning mode, and the means for obtaining changes furnish a behavior model for groups in the process of change. If an authority figure resists changes, and if subterfuge, underground tactics, deviousness, and dishonesty are used to obviate the authority structure, the planned changes will contain the same group tactics; thus the seeds of failure for the new attainments are sown.

3. *Participation in change is a voluntary commitment as is opposition to change, and the battle must be freely and overtly fought.* The implications of this condition are (1) that the only pressures existing on individual participants are peer group pressures and (2) that only in discussions where differences are aired openly without authority pressure for a particular previously determined outcome can there be true resolution through the examination of available alternatives. In addition, mutual agreement must be reached within the change group and not imposed by an authority figure.

4. *All relevant or interdependent units are involved or oriented to the fact that the process of change is occurring in one of the groups so that changes do not damage, shock, or interrupt other contingent units.* For instance, if nurses wish to change the delivery pattern in a section of an agency to make their care better quality, nurses of other sections, physicians, other departments—such as, x-ray, lab, and dietary—and all authority people involved should be notified so that shock, threat, and articulation problems are anticipated and minimized. Organizational patterns undergoing change in a nursing care situation need to be communicated to other departments interconnected with nursing so that others can aid the changes instead of blocking them, and so that the changes do not interrupt or decrease the effectiveness of others or services to the client. The administration could question the feasibility or workability of the new plan or the plan could fail, not because the changes are ineffective but because the proper "other" people were not consulted, alerted, oriented, or included in the planning phase.

PREDICTIVE PRINCIPLE: *Group commitment to the change process itself instead of specific changes enables continuing investigation, growth, and improvement.*

Groups who organize for change and who proceed to plan and implement change can devise a desired change that gets frozen into decisions of total commitment. Commitment to the specific change, rather than to changing, is a trap. Using words like "provisional," "tentative," "trial," and "interim" communicates the concept of change as a process—continuing and progressing forever. Nurse commitment to flexibility, innovation, and creativity becomes real only with use. The process-of-change concept is actualized by building a framework for change that provides for and necessitates constant use of feedback for making continuous alterations to the whole nursing care system. For instance, no public health nurse would make a plan for a visit that was acted upon regardless of the conditions encountered on the visit. The conditions encountered upon arriving at the client's home would become rapidly gathered feedback that would probably be utilized quickly to alter the preconceived plan. The same habit of gathering and utilizing feedback and altering plans becomes an activity habit, whether one is dealing with nursing care delivery system, individual patient care, or organizational structure.

BASIC ORGANIZATIONAL PATTERNS FOR CHANGING

Most health agencies are organized for stability. Standing committees, steering committees, executive committees, and ad hoc committees are the avenues through which the work of the agency is accomplished. Normal bureaucratic agencies are structured to change slowly. They do change, but their response to the forces causing the need to change is slowed by the very mechanisms that provide them with stability and permanency. To speed change to make agencies more responsive to social forces, new, sometimes temporary and sometimes permanent alterations must be made in the organizational structure.

PREDICTIVE PRINCIPLE: *Use of an organizational pattern for changing that utilizes a theoretical framework for guiding the logistics of human resources in a task-oriented system promotes effective and efficient use of energy toward attainment of the goal.*

Organizations can take a variety of organizational patterns or structures. The types described here will be traditional (bureaucratic) nursing agency organization, modified traditional or "linking pin," collegia, and functional team.

Traditional or bureaucratic systems are typical of nursing service organizations. Hospitals, colleges, most businesses, and governmental agencies in the United States function under a hierarchial structure. Committee structure pyramids toward the top chaironeships, which are awarded by rank and tenure. A committee superstructure of "chairpersons" meet and plan the work other committees are to do. Fig. 7 illustrates this organizational format. Changes are slow and difficult to make when using this organizational pattern. Response time is delayed while decisions are filtered through a maze of official channels.

Nursing organizations usually have all six characteristics listed by Bennis as typical of authoritarian organizations[*]:

1. They have a division of work based on functional specialization (often medical model clinical specialization).
2. They have clear-cut channels of communications and hierarchy of authority and responsibility.
3. They are characterized by rules and by laws and job descriptions that cover the rights, duties, responsibilities, and relationships of members.

---

[*]Bennis, W. G.: Changing organizations, New York, 1966, McGraw-Hill Book Co., p. 5.

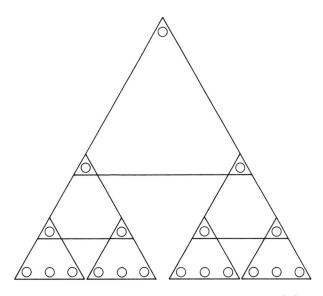

Fig. 7. Traditional pyramid type committee structure of bureaucracies.

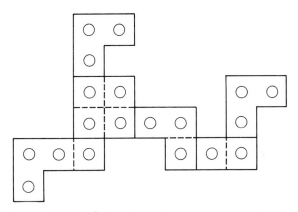

Fig. 8. Linking pin organizational structure. One person on a given task group serves on another task group working on a related task, thus furnishing a communication link and enabling the tasks to complement each other.

4. They have specific and predetermined procedural specifications and directions for handling work situations.
5. There is a certain amount of impersonality in the relationships between levels of the hierarchy.
6. Tenure and promotion are based on job or technical competence.

The modified traditional or "linking pin" organizational system has many of the characteristics of the preceding list. It varies somewhat in that the groups within the organization have some autonomy; leaders may be appointed or elected and are not necessarily chosen because they are ranking members of the hierarchy; leadership can rotate periodically, and one or more members of each group belong either to another group or to a central "executive or ad-

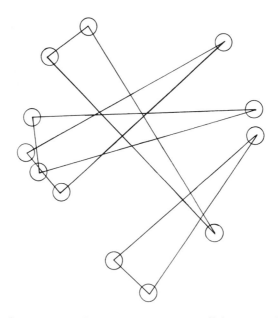

Fig. 9. Collegia. Objectives are clear cut. Participants collaborate with whom they need to at the time to achieve the goal. Lines are temporal. Membership in group is by ability. (From Bevis, E. O.: Curriculum building in nursing: a process, St. Louis, 1973, The C. V. Mosby Co.)

visory" board or group, thus linking each group and providing continuity, liaison, and communication. Procedure manuals, job descriptions, and other marks of bureaucratic organization are still in evidence. However, in linking pin organizational structure, committees are small, task oriented, and organized so that one member of a task committee serves on a related committee and is the communications pathway that enables work to be complementary and supportive toward goal attainment. Authority persons may or may not be the "link" (see Fig. 8).

On the opposite side of the continuum is a very loosely knit organizational pattern called a collegia. Individual accountability is an earmark of a collegial organization; roles are almost completely blurred and can shift and change with the task to be accomplished (see Fig. 9). Small groups assemble and shift in membership based upon the needs of the group to accomplish an objective. Group membership is temporal as is group leadership. Leadership is almost always by ability to facilitate the task, knowledge of the part of the task being worked upon, sudden inspiration or insights, and other phenomena. Investment of energy is toward the task, and no energy is committed to stabilizing the group. The "job" or "task" to be accomplished can be envisioned as being like a basketball passed back and forth among the players according to their place on the court, the pattern of play, or their particular talents. The group moves the ball down the court throwing it from one person or small group to another until at last someone puts it in the basket and the job is finished. If the ball hits the backboard, bounces back into play (feedback), reworking occurs until the ball is finally put through the basket and the goal is attained.

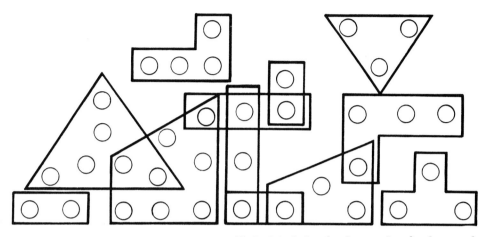

Fig. 10. Functional team. Groups are established and dissolved around tasks that need doing. Membership is by ability to contribute to the task. Role blurring occurs. Rank, position, and tenure are unimportant. All participate equally. (From Bevis, E. O.: Curriculum building in nursing: a process, St. Louis, 1973, The C. V. Mosby Co.)

The type of organization that offers the most for change in nursing is a modification and synthesis of the collegia and linking pin approaches—the functional team or task group organization.

In functional teams (see Fig. 10), groups or task forces of from two to five participants are organized around specific tasks. Membership on the task force lasts for the duration of the job. Once the job is accomplished, the task force dissolves. Role blurring occurs, and task force members contribute on equal footing according to their ability to contribute. Leadership in the group evolves from group needs and is not imposed on the group from without. Ground rules may change from task to task or from day to day within the same task force, for they too are generated in response to the needs of the task and not on a permanent basis. Completed work can either be sent to another task group for a critique—called an alter group or a feedback group (see Fig. 11)—or be submitted to the whole group. Reworking, revising, or altering based upon the feedback may be done by the same task force or may be altered by the critiquing group depending upon the agreement between the groups.

BASIC PLANNING STRATEGIES FOR CHANGING

An altered organization pattern for change preserves an altered way of looking at the task of changing. Often nursing care groups do not know what they wish to change to. They just know what they wish to change from. The goals and the content of changing can be separated from the process of changing. The change process can follow any number of patterns. The most effective pat-

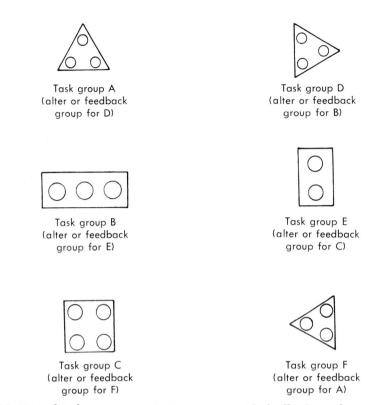

Fig. 11. Typical task group organization pattern with feedback or alter group assignments. (From Bevis, E. O.: Curriculum building in nursing: a process, St. Louis, 1973, The C. V. Mosby Co.)

terns use a task analysis framework. Task analysis is a methodology that arose from systems analysis. Systems analysis was used during World War II to ensure the delivery of weapons to the fighting forces by specific times. Systems analysis has been most commonly associated with the space program and has been highly successful in enabling many companies manufacturing a small component of a space system to complete their work and deliver their component at the time specified with confidence that the component would work effectively when interlinked with the other components being produced. These same methods are now being used by agencies to produce change. The change process is analyzed into component tasks. These tasks are then assigned to small groups. The completed product is used as a basis for the next stage of work forming a systemic linkage toward goals.

PREDICTIVE PRINCIPLE: *An explicit and definitive task analysis supports the ability of the client system to have an overall view of the subgoals and tasks to accomplish these goals.*

PREDICTIVE PRINCIPLE: *Formation and assignment of task groups according to the task, time limitations and capabilities of the change participants enables each member to contribute optimally.*

PREDICTIVE PRINCIPLE: *Organization of change participants around components of task analysis decreases "power" focus and increases goal orientation of work groups.*

The traditional way of organizing for change involves the establishment of committees. Committees, subcommittees, and ad hoc committees are the modes used in most bureaucratic organizations that rely on parliamentary law, parliamentary procedures, and parliamentary organizational forms. Committees have several characteristics that make them poor means for achieving change.

1. Committees tend to be power bases for individuals and factions in an organization. Much effort then goes into maintaining the power group, obtaining more power, and exercising power.
2. Power struggles tend to develop over traditional "red flag" issues, and individuals lock into a win-lose situation. The parliamentary procedures then tend to inhibit the search for alternatives that are win-win. The very act of voting locks people into win-lose modes.
3. Once power struggles arise in a committee and power lines are drawn, each new issue perpetuates the power struggle. This causes compromises to be made in ways that may pull the teeth from changes. This is done over the issue of power and influence and not often over the issue.
4. Committee membership becomes a prestige item, and changes that threaten the prestige, power, or existence of membership are resisted. Thus the committee tends to structure to perpetuate its own existence. Energy that could go into accomplishing goals is funneled off into committee maintenance.

The first major planning strategy for change is to opt for a structure that enables nurses and interested others to form small loosely knit task groups. These groups are formed of individuals who have an interest in or expertise for a specific task to achieve a specific goal. A task group organizational pattern assumes a task analysis format. Task analysis is a method of taking a large goal or "piece" of desired change and breaking it down into the steps, subgoals, or "tasks" that will ensure the reaching of the overall objective. Often the sheer size and magnitude of a change is frightening. Task analysis is reassuring in that groups can see the probability of succeeding in a small given task, where the overall job may be overwhelming. Small tasks or jobs are easier to achieve, and success is fairly quick, clear, and definitive. Success then breeds successes, and the reinforcement of completing one small bit of the total job motivates and energizes the nursing group to go on to the next task group and the next task. New people, new working relationships, and a new task dissipate the potential for developing power plays that siphon energy from the job to be done.

Every change goal can be reached by the simple expedient measure of analyzing the steps necessary to reach the goal. In each of the steps or sequence components there is a group of tasks for that component that must occur before that phase of development can be successfully organized and accomplished. Each group will need to analyze the tasks that are necessary to the change patterns of each individual nursing group. The following is an example of a task analysis.

Example of a task analysis

GOAL: To create a better nursing care record or charting form and system

TASK ANALYSIS:

1. Devise criteria for a desirable charting form.
2. Imagine components of a format that would meet those criteria.
3. Generate two or three alternative plans for using the components.
4. Choose a plan or synthesize from the ones presented.
5. Measure synthesized plan against established criteria.
6. Plan and select ways and means for testing a sample run of the new charting forms.
7. Institute the test run.
8. Get feedback from testers and share with all work groups.
9. Alter plan, using feedback.
10. Retest.
11. Confirm and implement, or revise and retest the plan until perfected.
12. Establish regular evaluation and review so change is ongoing.

EXAMPLE OF TASK ANALYSIS FOR SUBGOAL 1: Devise criteria for a desirable charting form.

1. Survey target group: What do participants like about present forms? What is disliked about them? What would the members prefer in a form? Categorize and sort findings and provide summary.
2. Survey like agencies over the country for sample forms and analyze for strengths and limitations. Categorize and sort findings; provide a summary.
3. Survey the literature on nursing record formats. Distribute useful articles or annotated notes or summaries to target group.
4. Get summaries and findings from all task groups. Ask three different task groups working independently to present the criteria by which they would evaluate a charting form and system.
5. Each of the three groups presents its criteria to three different alter groups for critique and feedback.
6. Selects and uses the feedback felt appropriate to improve criteria.
7. Present criteria of all three task groups to the target population. Get feedback and suggestions.
8. One task group uses feedback to make one criteria list for use in creating a charting form and system.

The task force organizational pattern allows implementation of a format for change that facilitates optimal participation by all people involved in change. A task analysis framework for organizing nursing care systems change enables tasks small enough to be handled in a short time span to be assigned to a specific group for a specific purpose.

Power struggles have little time to develop, and compromise is often delayed until adequate numbers of alternatives have been generated. Groups are small enough so that each member can generate possibilities and alternatives and bring them to the group for a critique. The group can then put together the desired product from individual contributions.

Task groups are transitory, membership expectations are for a temporal existence, work is task oriented with no energy given to maintaining the group, and dissolution is natural when the task is completed.

Working in task groups using a task analysis as a basis for organizing for change accomplishes some of the following:

1. Explicit and definitive task analysis provides client systems with an overall view of goals and steps that must be taken to reach the goals.
2. Established target dates enable change participants to pace their work realistically.
3. Temporal organization keeps the faculty and students job or task oriented and decreases focus on power.
4. Participating in task groups outside the area of immediate skill widens the horizon of individual members' views of nursing, decreases tunnel vision, provides scope, and brings fresh ideas from people not necessarily "locked into" a single system or way of accomplishing a goal or viewing a concept.
5. Working with people outside of usual committee structure broadens the base of working relationships and decreases fantasies about what colleagues are like; it establishes new communication habits and patterns.

PREDICTIVE PRINCIPLE: *Feedback from an alter group during the planning phase increases the probability that the group product will meet the staff needs, fulfill the task charge, and be useful to the target system.*

The second planning strategy that is most useful is to provide for feedback prior to total faculty consideration. Feedback is provided by task groups called alter groups (see Fig. 11). These critique groups provide checks and balances so that the creators of an idea, or task, can have the benefit of objective feedback, for example, noninvolved eyes for examining the work, asking questions, suggesting clarification or elucidation of specific parts, looking at congruencies between parts, suggesting revision, addition, or deletion in the work, and any other functions of feedback. The use of an alter group not only improves the product of the task group and helps to prepare it for total group discussion, it also widens the base of support through investment. When the second group becomes involved, they have already participated in the accomplishing of the task and therefore are prepared to speak to it and to support, at least in some measure, the group originally assigned to that task. The more people participate in the creation of an idea or the completion of a task, the more balanced the discussion of that suggested alternative is likely to be.

PREDICTIVE PRINCIPLE: *Generating several alternative solutions to a problem to achieve a goal enables the group to select an alternative most nearly in keeping with group needs.*

The third basic planning strategy suggested here is the generation of more than one alternative for every phase of, or task in, change building (see example task analysis). Choice is perhaps the most important aspect of facilitating change. And one of the reasons preplanned change can be so effective is that groups need not be faced with having to take an alternative because it is the only one available. Group planning for change includes, at every phase, the assigning of more than one task group to a task, with directions to work independently of each other, and the offering of more than one alternative plan to the total group. The consequences of having a choice are (1) groups tend to be more stimulated as they look at alternatives and discuss the potentialities and liabilities of each plan; (2) congruence or incongruence of parts of the plans with the theoretical base of the total plan are brought to light; and (3) the best parts of the alternatives can be pooled for developing a plan that meets the needs of the group.

PREDICTIVE PRINCIPLE: *Explicit rewards or recognition of individual or group achievement reinforces changing behaviors and promotes continuing efforts toward realization of goals.*

The last important strategy for change to be discussed here involves an obvious and explicit reward system. There is reward inherent in creating workable changes, which are tangible manifestations of visions. The more emphasis that can be placed upon the continuity of the road from the past (what individuals wished to accomplish) to the present (what the total group has accomplished), the greater will be the feeling of success. Beyond the reinforcement of accomplishing goals is the individual group member's contribution to that goal. Often work becomes such a synthesis of so many people's ideas that individual contributions are lost, and an anonymity develops that makes the work itself impersonal and easy to disown as not being a part of each person as an individual. There are some things that change agents can do to keep the personal element in the changes without destroying the group feeling. For instance, when a task group of three or four people collaborate on a special project and generate a piece of the puzzle that is particularly fitting for distribution to others or for publication, it is reinforcing to give recognition to the people preparing the product. By-lines, such as "prepared by Dianne Nicholson and Lucy Miller, in collaboration with other members of the nursing staff of Hillview Health Center," are expressive of the individual work, and the contribution of the "whole," and thus give special credit to the authors without detracting from the general credit due the group. Following are other reinforcing activities:

1. Encourage and facilitate publication of materials generated.
2. Provide letters, encouragement, and active support for efficiency evaluations and promotions.
3. Speak of specific contributions individuals have made to "power" people, for example, head nurses, supervisors, and other administrators.
4. Promote publicity for innovative endeavors through local newspapers, agency newsletters, and so on.
5. Celebrate milestones of accomplishment with small parties (this activity interrupts flow and marks progress and thus provides a point of reference).
6. Save early work as a starting point marker to make comparisons and provide perspectives on how far the group has come in building changes.

7. Distribute general congratulatory letters periodically when particularly effective results have been achieved.

These activities are useful for role modeling the process of valuing the contributions of individuals. Too often nurses tend to devalue their own work and value that of outsiders. Any activity that provides patterns of behavior establishing the value of "home town prophets" builds self-confidence and helps the group make it legitimate to use each other as consultants.

APPLICATION OF PREDICTIVE PRINCIPLES OF CHANGING

A representative from the evening shift approaches the head nurse and states: "The afternoon personnel have asked me to represent them. They wish to discontinue charting on evening shift patients. It is a meaningless bit of busy work and a waste of time. We could just check off medications and sign the nursing record page that we've seen the patient."

PROBLEM	PRINCIPLES	PRESCRIPTION
How to enable the group to determine what changes in charting and charting policies will best meet the needs of patients and staff.	Failure of a nursing care delivery system to meet the needs of its practitioners, clients, and/or employers ensures changes in or the death of the system.	Make critique of the system legitimate and elicit consensus that change is needed.
	The breakdown of effectiveness of standard procedures and traditional organization causes an increase in anxiety of the individual nursing care giver.	Elicit agreement to participate in work toward finding workable solution to problem.
	Experiencing high anxiety levels provides a need for change or adaptation accompanied by an increase in individual and collective energy.	Channel energy into task groups, goal setting, and attainment.
	Need for change or adaptation stimulates personal fantasies of solutions or anticipation of the achievement of objectives.	Involve group in brainstorming about problems and possible workable nursing recording forms and procedures.
	Free exchange of ideas about goals and subgoals enables the establishment of specific and legitimate goals and collaboration for their achievement.	Brainstorm about a process for change that would involve all concerned and accomplish goals; brainstorm about goals and steps or tasks necessary to achieve goals.
	Explicit participation and support of the administration for changes ensures the changing group has the power and authority to implement plans for change.	Invite appropriate power people to take part in the discussions from the first or have regular appointments; be sure power people condone or consent to potential change.
	Creating environmental and operational conditions that nurture the change process sup-	

Continued.

PROBLEM	PRINCIPLES	PRESCRIPTIONS
	ports the potential success of the change effort.	
	Use of an organizational pattern for changing that utilizes a theoretical framework for guiding the logistics of human resources in a task-oriented system promotes effective and efficient use of energy toward attainment of the goal.	Get consensus for an organization for change that uses everyone's potential without regard to status, rank, or position—transient task groups of some kind.
	An explicit and definitive task analysis supports the ability of the client system to have an overall view of the sub-goals and tasks to accomplish these goals.	Assign a task group to do a task analysis on overall goal.
	Formation and assignment of task groups according to the task, time limitations, and capabilities of the change participants enables each member to contribute optimally.	Assign task groups to tasks identified by the above group.
	Feedback from an alter group during the planning phase increases the probability that the group product will meet the staff needs, fulfill the task charge, and be useful to the target system.	When tasks are completed, give to feedback group; rework task, based on feedback.
	Generating several alternative solutions to a problem to achieve a goal enables the group to select an alternative most nearly in keeping with group needs.	Be sure that several task groups work on alternative solutions so group will have a choice.
	Explicit rewards or recognition of individual or group achievement reinforces changing behaviors and promotes continuing efforts toward realization of goals.	Acknowledge groups' and participants' contribution; write notes for change participants; acknowledge ideas; give reinforcement for participation; set up mechanism for continued reviewing, testing, and evaluating of planned program of change.

BIBLIOGRAPHY

BOOKS

Alexander, E. L.: Nursing administration in the hospital health care system, St. Louis, 1972, The C. V. Mosby Co.

Bennis, W. G.: Changing organizations, New York, 1966, McGraw-Hill Book Co.

Bennis, W. G. Benne, K. D., and Chin, R.: The planning of change, ed. 2, New York, 1969, Holt, Rinehart and Winston, Inc.

Bevis, E. O.: Curriculum building in nursing: a process, St. Louis, 1973, The C. V. Mosby Co.

Havelock, R. G.: A guide to innovation in education, Ann Arbor, Mich., 1970, Center for Research on Utilization of Scientific Knowledge, Institute of Social Research, The University of Michigan Press.

Saunders, L.: Permanence and change. In Lewis, E. P.: Changing patterns of nursing practice, New York, 1971, The American Journal of Nursing Co.

Seiler, J. A.: Systems analysis in organizational behavior, Homewood, Ill., 1967, The Dorsey Press, Inc.

PERIODICALS

Simms, L. L.: Administrative changes and implications for nursing practice in the hospital, Nurs. Clin. North Am. 8(2):227-234, June, 1973.

CHAPTER SEVEN

Predictive principles of leadership behavior

FUNDAMENTALS OF LEADERSHIP

Understanding various managerial systems and the work environment provides the leader with a basis for determining a suitable type of leadership for the situation or for developing congruent adaptive behaviors within the environment.

A clear operational definition of leadership expectations expedites role definition and role enactment.

Knowledge of theory levels and ability to formulate valid predictive principles promote the leader's ability to identify the levels on which members are functioning to facilitate growth in problem solving and goal attainment.

Identification of leadership characteristics associated with managerial climates facilitates the conversion of characteristics into operational behaviors.

AWARENESS OF SELF

Knowledge and understanding of factors that contribute to mental health permit personal assessment of one's own state of mental health.

Identification of the leader's own needs aids in the identification of needs of others.

Accurate appraisal of self promotes healthy emotional organization.

Acceptance of self creates a climate for the acceptance of others.

KNOWLEDGE OF THE JOB

The demands of the situation in which a leader is to function influence the qualities, characteristics, knowledge, and skills necessary for successful leadership.

The degree to which the leader is clinically knowledgeable and competent directly influences feelings of security about the appropriateness of nursing activity.

MUTUAL RESPECT

Understanding and practicing the basic elements of mutual respect facilitate effective leadership.

Expressions of respect for others by the leader precipitate acts of mutual respect among members.

OPEN CHANNELS OF COMMUNICATION

Knowledge of appropriate channels of communication facilitates efficient utilization of line organization.

The nurse working in an expanded role provides leadership initiative in establishing channels of communication congruent with the role.

KNOWLEDGE OF PARTICIPANT'S CAPABILITIES

An understanding of sociocultural backgrounds of members assists the leader to make an assessment of job capabilities.

Reactions to stress influence efficiency of performance in the work situation.

Knowledge of a care giver's preparation and experience promotes fullest use of skills and provides a basis for continued growth.

ENVIRONMENT

A work environment that is open and amenable to valid change assists in personal and professional growth and development.

The practice of professional nursing carries with it the responsibility to lead, manage, and/or facilitate others. Effective leadership is a learned process; it is the ability to mobilize behaviors toward the achievement of a purpose through the investiture and acceptance of authority. The culmination of all nursing activity is in the delivery of patient care. Scientifically based, problem-oriented behavior in the client's interest will produce quality care and is likely to be administered at less cost to the consumer of health services.

The outcome of nursing leadership function is some aspect of nursing practice. Administrative emphasis is on clinical competency, proficiency in nursing performance, management of clinical nursing activities and patient advocacy, as well as on the operation of a unit. Health care delivery groups with varying responsibilities for patient care need to interact with each other for better patient care in a systematic and collaborative fashion. Communication between administration, medicine, other health care givers, consumers, and nurses concerning health care will increase the effectiveness of that care. The overall quality of patient care is effective and efficient only to the degree that nurse-leaders relate to the environment in which they perform in a significant and organizational manner.

This chapter discusses the fundamentals of leadership, awareness of self, and the knowledge of the tasks to be performed. Similarly, it is concerned with the capabilities of the leader, as well as with the environment in which nursing care is rendered. Most of these concepts have been integrated into the content of the preceding chapters.

FUNDAMENTALS OF LEADERSHIP

Historically, leadership was awarded to the strong. From primitive man to the present, rule of the powerful has been felt on all levels. Cunning and brain power have replaced brute strength, but the system still exists in some milieus. It is a hallmark of an advanced civilization that leaders receive their authority from the groups they lead and maintain their leadership only so long as they meet the needs of the groups they are guiding.

Even in the most democratic of leadership situations, power struggles exist. In nursing, for example, for too long the capable nurse-leaders have not been delegated authority commensurate with responsibility for planning and decision making. Traditional management practices reflect the belief that nurses at the operational level require close supervision and control; therefore, someone else must retain the power. The devestment of authority from those nurses on operational levels has led to power struggles. If ignored, these power struggles dissipate energy, divide and demoralize the participants, and result in decreased productivity.

There are three generally accepted categories of leadership: autocratic, democratic, and laissez-faire. Autocratic leadership means that one person has supreme power to make decisions for others. Democratic leadership means authority is vested in the leader by the group, and the group has a part in decision making. Laissez-faire leadership means that group members do as they please, and neither the group members nor the leader accepts the responsibility for decision making.

One category of leadership is rarely practiced alone. Combinations of different categories are used depending on the situation, the group, and the characteristics of the leader. A leader tends to practice a given category of leadership dictated by his personality, background, experience, and knowledge and the context of the nursing situations. The old axiom "leaders are born, not made" is not true. Leadership is learned. The nurse can acquire leadership ability through the educational process and by the consistent application of appropriate principles to everyday nursing situations.

PREDICTIVE PRINCIPLE: *Understanding various managerial systems and the work environment provides the leader with a basis for determining a suitable type of leadership for the situation or for developing congruent adaptive behaviors within the environment.*

Autocratic leadership

Autocratic (authoritarian) leadership is a directive style of supervision. Common characteristics found in autocracy are a low degree of participation by the people involved, a high degree of punitiveness, a high degree of pressure placed on the worker for output of work, much emphasis on structure and policy, and minimal emphasis on consideration, mutual trust, respect, or warmth for the employee. The focus is upon working, with greater emphasis upon the system than upon the client. Decisions are made by the leader, or responsibility for making them is delegated by him.

Autocratic leadership is the traditional forte of nursing. Historically, the chain of command from supervisor, head nurse, staff nurse, senior student, to the beginning student carried with it status that commanded awe of and unquestioning obedience to those in charge. In this organizational structure the doctor was omnipotent, and the existence of nurse functions based upon nursing knowledge and independent of physicians' orders was all but unrecognized. The subservient attitude exemplified by "I'm not paid to think, I'm paid to follow orders" marked this type of organization. Decisions were made by designated people, and few dared question their authority. The autocratic leader speaks in terms of *I, me, my,* and *mine* even when referring to group effort. *We, us,* and *our* seem lost from his vocabulary. Individualism is sacrificed for the sake of organizational goals.

The autocrat is stern, strict, or just, according to his own established principles and guidelines for action. He gives praise or criticism to each member on his own initiative and remains aloof from people most of the time. His principles and guidelines may be effective, but they may not be in the best interest of the individuals involved. He has no one to turn to for validation; therefore, since the autocratic leader makes all decisions and plots all directives, he retains all authority, as well as all responsibility. Since there is minimal group participation, there is limited commitment to the results of group behavior, little feeling of responsibility for the success or failure of the enterprise, and always there is someone else for the group to blame—the leader or another scapegoat.

Authoritarian leadership implies frustration of significant needs in the followers. Because there is no safe outlet for the expression of feelings, morale and sometimes productivity are lowered, and reactions of hostility, apathy, or blind obedience can occur. The led are usually unwilling to exercise initiative, in fear that innovation will increase the chance for error and will result in punitive measures. In terms of service to clients, the followers tend to seek satisfaction from the abstract values of the enterprise, such as monetary remuneration or promotion, rather than from the value of service to people.

When nurses in practice situations have fixed rules established for them and feel they have no recourse, one avenue of retaliation is to comply with the demands made upon them but to retreat personally. Apathy spreads throughout the membership, resulting in demoralization, decreased effectiveness, and poor care for the patients.

Blind obedience to autocracy may result because some nurses prefer to be followers, they fear responsibility, or they have other interests or needs that take precedence over the job at hand. They take the path of least resistance on the job because their energies are expended elsewhere. Other nurses may believe they do not possess the qualities necessary for leadership and are satisfied to function under others. Some nurses, however, modify the environment in ways that allow them to be effective regardless of bureaucratic leadership.

Laissez-faire leadership

Laissez-faire leadership is described as open and permissive, abdicating, frustrating, confusing, and uncontrolled. Laissez-faire leadership is leadership in which each group member sets goals independently. It is the least efficient of the three types of leadership and exists either in rebellion against autocratic leadership or because no leader is invested with responsibility and no one assumes the role. It exists when a leader is too weak or too threatened to exercise the functions of leadership or when lack of trust within the group prevents unity. Hostility generated by autocratic leadership can produce a nurse who is determined to be the opposite of all that was despised in the autocratic system and thereby withholds leadership activities and functions Laissez-faire.

Because of lack of information, this nurse practices laissez-faire leadership in the mistaken belief that democratic rule is being practiced. Guidelines, rules and regulations, limit setting, and decisions are not seen as safeguards for the individual group member, the patient, and the agency but as infringements on the rights and dignity of the worker.

The staff nurse who has great need of approval may practice laissez-faire leadership out of fear of offending group members. This leader wants to please everyone and, in the attempt, fails to give strength and direction, to set limits, and to conduct open and honest discussions.

Democratic leadership

Democratic leadership is employed with the consent and support of those who are led. The leader's security does not depend on the maintenance of the existing conditions. A democratic climate is conducive to the process of exploration and discovery of the individual. People sense that their own feelings and thoughts, as well as those of others, are important. Democracy is authority invested in the leader by individuals or a group, with the right to make certain decisions and judgments and to take action. Democracy does not mean an investment of *all* power in the leader, nor does it imply that a vote is taken on everything.

Democracy is the power to act sometimes in behalf of others. In this system it is legitimate to express controversial beliefs and to give and receive feedback so that behaviors may be altered. Ultimately, in the democratic system the leader may be stripped of the power invested in him by the group. In other instances, channels of administration can be bypassed. Jeffersonian democracy is classless. Each individual has equal rights and opportunities to become the leader; thus leadership exists on all levels.

Inherent in democracy is the major element of *trust*, confidence by the group that the leader will function in the best interest of all concerned—client, community, the nursing group, and agency—and by the leader that the membership will support him.

For trust and support to exist, both leader and members must possess successful experiences in having their needs and expectations met by each other. Free and open communications using appropriate channels can promote a feeling of security; the leader is confident in his ability to work with people and resources available to him for the benefit of his clients. He accepts responsibility for his failures rather than projecting them onto individuals or an organization. Because he knows his only limitation to be his level of competence, he is committed to growth as a professional. Assessment of each care giver's ability and optimal use of his knowledge and skills will develop individual and group potential to the maximum. Within the democratic framework, meaningful goals can be established and the participants can develop ways for objectively evaluating their own accomplishment.

It is not possible to specify the type of management that will be most productive in any given situation. The democratic approach is proposed as the ideal method of operation, but occasions will arise when the authoritarian or even the laissez-faire approach will be desirable. In most instances leadership style is a mixture of the three types of leadership. For nursing, autocracy modified by some democratic operations is the general rule.

PREDICTIVE PRINCIPLE: *A clear operational definition of leadership expectations expedites role definition and role enactment.*

Nursing leadership is the ability to use the processes of life to facilitate the movement of a person, a group, a family, or a community toward the establishment and attainment of a goal (see Chapter 1). The strength of the leader's influence depends on the interactive variables of the task, the clients to be served, the organizational structure, the external environment, and the characteristics of the leader and the followers. Leadership is a learned behavior pattern; therefore, utilizing leadership role enactment theories is necessary for operationalizing the leadership process.

Critical attention should be given to the selection of nurse-leaders who are best able to learn and systematically utilize sound principles in problem solving. This problem-solving behavior will equip the nurse-leader to cope with the ever changing processes in the health scene as administrator, nurse clinician, counselor, teacher, and resource person whenever and whomever they serve.

PREDICTIVE PRINCIPLE: *Knowledge of theory levels and ability to formulate valid predictive principles promote the leader's ability to identify the levels on which members are functioning to facilitate growth in problem solving and goal attainment.*

The formulation of a valid theory is described fully in Chapter 1. Level I is composed of *naming,* or *labeling,* and *classifying,* or *categorizing,* the result. Level II also has two phases: *depicting,* or describing, and *factor relating.* The third level is *situation relating,* concerned with causal relationships. The fourth level in theory building is *situation producing,* comprised of the formulation of prescriptive theories. When situation-producing theories are analyzed, they consist of three aspects: (1) a definable goal, (2) a prescription, and (3) study or diagram of specific activities and directions, which if followed, produce a predicted result or attain preset goals. The final component in the fourth level is a survey list of resources, techniques, and behavioral patterns that can be structured into goal-producing activities. At this stage, the wider the nurse-leader's knowledge of experiences of related situations, treatments, and results produced, the more reliable the results. In addition, the nurse's behaviors will reflect more effectively the acquired principles or predictive theories, which predict desired outcomes. This knowledge of theory levels equips the leader with the tools necessary for identifying the level at which individuals and groups are operating and to provide guidance that will promote growth up through the levels.

PREDICTIVE PRINCIPLE: *Identification of leadership characteristics associated with managerial climates facilitates the conversion of characteristics into operational behaviors.*

A leadership characteristic is an attribute, quality, trait, or distinguishing mark of an individual. Leadership characteristics also imply a distinctive temperament or mood and include that which is outstanding in one's personality. This may be physical, mental, or social. A physical characteristic can be described as a peculiarity or walk or posture that sets the individual apart and makes him unique. It may also become an idiosyncrasy or a mannerism.

The use of climate in this book does not refer to temperature, such as humidity or other natural climatic conditions, but rather to the general context or overall picture of conditions in which one operates. Climate is thought of as a social condition or mood or a generality of opinion or attitude held by a group. This then becomes the climate of that group. In totality, climate includes opinions peculiar to a stated group of individuals or a society. One may speak of the social climate of a certain group as being warm or friendly. The converse is also true. The climate of a health agency may be open or closed toward those not initiated into the agency. For instance, those giving nursing care or medical treatment can create a climate of concern for the general welfare of the patient.

The following outline affords a partial comparative summary of the various climates that could exist in a health agency, divided into three major categories.

DEMOCRATIC	AUTHORITARIAN	LAISSEZ-FAIRE
Responsible and accountable	Accountable	Uncontrolled
Open	Defensive	Open
Facilitating	Restricting	Permissive
Freeing	Coercing	Abdicating
Encouraging	Discouraging	Frustrating
Accepting	Accepting and rejecting	Accepting and rejecting
Differences valued	Conforming valued	Indifferent
Variety	Uniformity	Variety
Equality	Inequality	Equality
Participative	Individual	Participative and individual
Self-legislative	Imposed legislation	Indifferent to legislation
Trusting	Fearing	Indifference
Available	Controlled availability	Available and unavailable
Encouraging	Forcing	Lacking in direction
Freedom of choice	Limited choice	Freedom of choice
Led by choice	Leader imposed	Led by choice
Cooperation	Competition	Confusion
Equal opportunity	Controlled opportunity	Open to opportunity
Opportunity	Exploitation	Uncontrolled
Challenge	Threat	Permissive
Recognition	Praise	Acceptance
Self-disciplined	Punishment	Lazy
Satisfaction	Reward	Acceptance

Leadership defined only by climate or characteristics becomes nonfunctional, as characteristics alone cannot be operationalized. Much research has been concerned with characteristics associated with the role of the leader. The successful administrator is commonly viewed as intelligent, possessing a well-balanced personality, assured of self-worth, accepting of others, a catalyst, responsible and accountable, having insight, imagination, and creativity, and as exercising good judgment in problem solving and decision making.

Characteristics and climate are not mutually exclusive; therefore neither operates alone. The climate around an individual does not remain constant, nor do his circumstances remain the same. It is not possible to say of a person that he "is always cooperative" or that he "is always permissive." Perhaps Leo Tolstoy best expresses the fluidity of man:

> One of the most widespread superstitions is that every man has his own special, definite qualities; that a man is kind, cruel, wise, stupid, energetic, apathetic, etc. Men are not like that. . . . Men are like rivers: the water is the same in each and alike in all; but every river is narrow here, is more rapid there, here slower, there broader, now clear, now cold, now dull, now warm. It is the same with men. Every man carries in himself the germs of every human quality, and sometimes one manifests itself, sometimes another, and the man often becomes unlike himself, while still remaining the same man.

Throughout life each individual establishes a definite life-style of his own. He develops response patterns that work best for him. The person will tend to repeat those experiences that bring satisfaction and to discard those that cause discomfort.

Employment of the trial and error method is a forfeiture or abdication of the leader's responsibility to deliberate choice in leadership. One must cognitively, consciously, and systematically develop those personal characteristics that will contribute to the advancement of the leadership role.

Characteristics, simply named, are in the first stage of theory building. They remain nonfunctional until they are developed through the theoretical pattern to actualization. To become effective or useful, each characteristic must be converted into behaviors that can be operationalized. For example, the leadership characteristic stated as "responsible" is described and depicted in the second level of theory as "functions within the framework of the employer or agency," "fulfills agreement for services," and "accounts for actions." The third level then is accepting responsibility for nursing care giving and promoting fulfillment of agreements made with clients for services. The fourth level of theory in actualizing leadership responsibility includes (1) assessment with client of his needs for care, (2) determination of alternatives, (3) identification of risks, (4) selection of alternatives for action, (5) establishment of schedule for implementation, (6) involvement of others, (7) setting criteria for evaluation, and (8) implementation.

AWARENESS OF SELF

Awareness of self is the ability to be sensitive to one's own needs, motives, and responses to stimuli. Self-awareness enables the nurse-leader to help followers understand themselves and to develop their potential. In turn, the more the nurse helps others to grow, the more self-growth will occur.

Traditionally, nurses are seen as self-sacrificing; their individual needs are viewed as unimportant. Even the struggle for economic security is more difficult because of the image of the nurse as a self-sacrificing and giving person. The nature of nursing draws people to the field who have a need to be useful to others. Recognition of the individual needs of nurses and finding ways to meet those needs free the nurse to meet the needs of the patient.

PREDICTIVE PRINCIPLE: *Knowledge and understanding of factors that contribute to mental health permit personal assessment of one's own state of mental health.*

The nurse enters the leadership role with certain needs, drives, and motives, and seeks satisfaction from the total work situation. Individual feelings are based on many variables dependent on goals and the nurse's ability to reach these goals. A person who follows a normal developmental pattern progresses from dependence (mother-child relationship) to the independent role and on to interdependence (in which a productive and satisfying working relationship with others is established). The basic urge of a human being is toward a state of physical, mental, and social well-being.

Insight—self-awareness—does not come in a vacuum; other people are involved in the process. In an environment where there is mutual respect, adequate feedback will take place and the leader will grow in self-awareness. The leader will then be able to carry out tasks of leadership in a better way and may achieve wholly unexpected and sometimes unique accomplishments.

PREDICTIVE PRINCIPLE: *Identification of the leader's own needs aids in the identification of needs of others.*

Man expresses needs from birth to death; the degree of importance of the need depends on conditions and circumstances. The basic needs are physiologic —the desire for food, rest, exercise, shelter, and protection from the elements. When basic needs are reasonably satisfied, others begin to motivate man, for he is not static. Other needs include the necessity for love, status, and recognition. The leader who understands his own needs in perspective and realizes that they are constantly changing can better understand these same needs in others.

PREDICTIVE PRINCIPLE: *Accurate appraisal of self promotes healthy emotional organization.*

PREDICTIVE PRINCIPLE: *Acceptance of self creates a climate for the acceptance of others.*

The leader's acceptance of himself enables him to accept his followers. Self-acceptance is built upon self-awareness; the leader who has achieved this status is likely to develop a sense of personal integrity and self-worth to the extent that he behaves constructively even when his authority is threatened. For example, when a care giver asks the leader, "Are you sure this is what we should do?" the leader may interpret the question as the follower's not feeling secure about the leader's judgement. The amount of anxiety the question creates and the leader's response depend on his self-image and self-awareness. If the nurse-leader believes the authority role is being questioned and feels threatened, he is apt to follow with a defensive response, such as "Don't you think I know what I'm doing?" or "What right have you to question my orders!" Such a response would bring about feelings of defense, hostility, and aggression in the questioner. If the nurse has insight and self-awareness, the focus of interaction can be on activities that will clarify messages and produce better results. The leader's response to the member might be, "Can you give me a better picture of your concern?" or "You don't feel comfortable about this plan of action?" The leader will then wait for the questioning person to elucidate his feelings. The results of this response are twofold: (1) the action in question will be reevaluated and (2) the nurse-leader will demonstrate acceptance of the member.

Self-understanding can be increased through evaluation of clinical conference processes. Members of the group can help the nurse-leader to expand self-understanding. Listening to tape recordings of meetings or conferences will help the nurse-leader develop insight and understanding regarding the effect of his behavior, attitudes, and methods on others. Assistance in the evaluative process can be sought from the group members involved.

Sensitivity training is another source of help to the nurse-leader. This training usually involves a series of meetings in which emphasis is placed on activities and interactions that develop greater awareness of a responsiveness to other's needs. The training group is designed to promote personal growth. It focuses on individual and group behavior, awareness of self, and social processes. The goal is to help members become more aware of the way they affect others and how others affect them, both consciously and unconsciously. Business and industry use this training extensively on the premise that leaders with greater insight into self have greater job potential and productivity.

Institutes and courses designed to assist in the development of increased self-understanding are often available to nurses through adult education programs, the community, professional groups, colleges and universities. Occasionally, highly qualified persons are willing to come to the agency if enough interest and action are generated. The nurse-leader can play an important role by becoming the facilitator and by requesting assistance in the task of self-development.

All methods for assisting the nurse-leader to increase self-understanding require an expenditure of time, effort, and money. The responsibility for seeking assistance lies with the recipient, but the provision of courses is an in-service educational activity.

If the nurse-leader is to develop to fullest maturity, avenues must be sought that assist in self-development. Just as cosmetics are used not because a woman is ugly but because she hopes that her best features will be accentuated and the less desirable ones will be subdued, the nurse seeks more complete self-understanding to minimize weaknesses and to maximize strengths.

The more the nurse knows about himself, the greater the likelihood of achieving healthy living. Attainment of conscious self-awareness is a difficult process. But personality may change, expand, and integrate even though the process is slow.

Every human being faces obstacles that thwart achievement of goals. The frustrations resulting from unsuccessful attempts to attain goals may elicit discomfort and feelings of inadequacy. When a goal is established, movement is in the direction of that goal. The individual tends to repeat those experiences that bring him satisfaction and to discard those that cause him discomfort. When an obstacle prevents goal achievement, aggressive reaction may occur either directly or indirectly. For example, a nurse-leader decides that a group meeting will be conducted to establish nursing care plans for the patients assigned. Plans for the meeting are announced to the group, and a time is set for early afternoon. During the course of the day, each of the members gives an excuse about why he cannot attend. The nurse-leader attempts to overcome the excuses but is alone at the time of the scheduled conference. The leader becomes frustrated and vents hostile feelings on the members throughout the remainder of the day. Nothing is accomplished except that the leader's reactions have been transmitted to others, who, in turn, act in the same nonconstructive manner.

The problem could have been resolved had the nurse identified feelings and attempted to determine the reasons for the resistance to the proposed conference. The most logical approach for gathering data in this situation is to ask those members involved the reasons for their resistance. At an ensuing session, the leader could raise the issue by reviewing the incident of the previous day. For instance: "I realize that I must have done something to cause all members to stay away, but I do not know what the mistake was. In order for me to avoid another incident of this kind, I need to know what I did. Will you help me?" or "Could you tell me more about it?" "What feelings led up to your action?" If the leader is sincere in desiring to learn the facts, the group members will recognize these feelings and honor them with feedback concerning the incident. Successes and failures can be validated so that similar incidents will not occur; the leader is then better equipped to move on toward desired goals.

Ideals of achievement are a part of human make-up. Many factors influence the development of concepts about what kind of person an individual would like to be. Ambitions, aspirations, satisfactions, and rewards change with each life experience. The nurse may have entered the profession because of a desire to help others, or he may have wished to become a specialist doing vital and exciting work. Either of the above ambitions may be achieved if the nurse assesses capabilities, recognizes limitations, and plans accordingly. For example, in the role of nurse-leader, planning, directing, and participating in the care giving process provides the leader a feeling of self-worth and satisfaction from being able to serve others and a perception of accomplishment from achieving a personal goal.

When a nurse's ability is inadequate for achievement of ambition, frustration occurs; if uninterrupted, it may destroy his sense of well-being. If knowledge and experience are insufficient for reaching goals, constructive steps must be taken to make up the inadequacies.

Self-confidence can be developed as increased self-knowledge is acquired and some successes are achieved. If the challenge of leading is too great for the nurse's capacity, lack of self-esteem and feelings of insecurity will arise. When the nurse-leader feels inadequate, such feelings may be the cause of destructive behavior; the leader may become too demanding and critical of others in an effort to maintain self-image. For example, the leader who feels incapable of understanding the cardiac monitoring system may assign a patient to be monitored to another nurse. When the nurse asks the leader for assistance in interpreting data, the leader may react with an angry statement, such as, "Don't you know what you are doing? A nurse should keep up with what is going on!" Thus the nurse-leader attempts to build self-esteem at the expense of another person.

The following would have been a constructive approach to the situation.

When the nurse-leader knew the group was to be responsible for the care of a patient requiring cardiac monitoring, the following steps could have been taken to ensure safety and high quality of care for the patient:

1. Making it known to the head nurse that no nurse member had the specialized knowledge required to assume care for a patient who required cardiac monitoring
2. Taking steps to secure a person qualified to care for such a patient
3. Initiating plans to gain the necessary knowledge

When the nurse becomes more understanding of his own assets and liabilities, develops a basic understanding of personal and professional self, and feels comfortable enough to share this knowledge with others, growth as a nurse-leader will occur.

KNOWLEDGE OF THE JOB

The nursing leadership role assumes certain basic knowledge and skills. These attributes are assured and perpetuated through accreditation of schools of nursing and hospitals, through the licensure of nurses, and through the system of rewards and punishments built into employment situations. Clients depend on the nurse's clinical judgment for giving the best possible service. The nurse-leader is expected to provide direction in all areas of planning, administering, and evaluating nursing care. The extent to which the nurse-leader is successful in role adaptation, perception, and response to leadership requirements directly relates to (1) the leader's ability to build theory and utilize it, (2) range of conscious role learning, (3) role taking, (4) role enactment, and (5) a large role repertoire.

PREDICTIVE PRINCIPLE: *The demands of the situation in which a leader is to function influence the qualities, characteristics, knowledge, and skills necessary for successful leadership.*

It is impossible for a nurse to possess knowledge and skills necessary to function in all aspects of nursing today, for this career is multifaceted and complex. But the practitioner can influence the development of optimal leadership abilities by collaborating with other persons to (1) preassess leadership qualities, characteristics, knowledge, and skills for the job, (2) plan ways and means to acquire additional service tools viewed as necessary for the proposed managerial role, (3) obtain feedback to ascertain increased level of competence, and (4) secure an assignment commensurate with knowledge and ability.

Clinical competence is effectively rewarded by advancement. Hence competent nurses are often assigned to cardinal positions. This clinical expertise contributes to effective guidance but does not ensure that the nurse will possess leadership qualities. The value of technical knowledge or proficiency in facilitating leadership depends on the situation and the tasks to be accomplished. If technical knowledge is not relevant to the goals established, it will be of minimal service either to the leader or to the recipient of services.

Anxiety is generated in situations that make demands for clinical knowledge the nurse has not acquired; this in turn disrupts organizational behavior patterns even in highly skilled nurses. All too often nurses are placed in roles where they are novices, in jobs that depend on knowledge pertaining to policy, procedure, and routine with which they are unfamiliar or that require expertise in unaccustomed clinical areas. This practice generates false incompetence. For example, a nurse-leader fully qualified to function in a pediatric unit may render poor service on an obstetrical unit. Clinical knowledge about separation anxiety in the 2-year-old child does not enable the nurse to make good judgments about post-partal bleeding.

Problems beyond the ability of the nurse-leader cause a high anxiety level and an indulgence in activities that in reality only drain off the excess energy generated by such high anxiety. An illustration of this is demonstrated by the following:

> A group is responsible for the care of an agitated patient who needs the constant presence of a care giver. The nurse-leader's energy and time are spent in trying to get the charge nurse to assign an extra person, attempting to get the nursing service office to send help, trying to get the physician to change his orders or to request a private duty nurse, or trying to get the patient transferred to a different unit or put into an isolated or maximum security room.

This nurse-leader spends time in fruitless efforts and activities that do not contribute to the solution of the problem. Admitting ignorance about the care of agitated patients would have damaged the leader's self-esteem; consequently, the nurse-leader avoided this by engaging in activities, such as trying to obtain aid, that were acceptable to the group. Any consequent difficulties with the agitated patient can conveniently be the fault of those who did not respond as requested.

The nurse who is secure and has the ability to care for this type of patient helps the care givers devise ways of handling this problem. This can be achieved through teaching those skills necessary to safely and effectively care for the patient and through planning a cooperative effort. The time and energy spent in teaching and planning for this emergency will profit the whole membership when a similar problem arises. Goal-directed activity generates self-confidence, which is transmitted to others and is reinforced by success.

Self-confidence is born of success and reinforced by enough success to allow failures to be perceived, not as basic inadequacies, but as momentary or transient failures. Self-confidence enables the nurse-leader to identify areas of knowledge and ignorance and to instigate activities that will increase knowledge and expand professional expertise.

Continuing education through self-study, in-service programs, or formal programs (organizations and colleges) will enable the nurse-leader to keep pace with professional technology. Part of the solution to the need for an increase in quality care is in utilization: better use of employees through on-the-job training for specialized skills. Policies that encourage continuing education will help to achieve the goals. Because of increased efficiency and fuller utilization of individual productivity potential, the professionally knowledgeable nurse is an economic asset to the public and to the employing agency.

The energy output utilized in attempting to circumvent a nursing situation decreases when the nurse can cope with a situation; energy can be directed toward achievement rather than circumvention.

The recent trend to offer nursing services at the colleague-peer relationship level, as with the primary care nurse who works in contractual agreement with the client, and other special nursing roles—described as extender, expander, assistant, associated, clinical specialist, and practitioner—necessitate preparation beyond that normally provided in nursing curricula.* Whatever the label and however the functions are described, an expanded role requires a corresponding increase in knowledge and skills to meet the challenge. Schools of nursing, particularly baccalaureate and graduate programs, are deluged with requests from federal, state, regional, and local commissions, as well as from individuals, to prepare the nurse with primary skills to provide better health care to increased numbers of people. Major content areas that have been largely absent from nursing curricula in the past are those of physical and developmental assessment and health history. For the practicing nurse, consistent acquisition of new knowledge requires aptitude and an investment of time and money. The nurse-leader committed to assuming a new role will seek and complete programs of study that will provide the necessary supplementary preparation.

PREDICTIVE PRINCIPLE: *The degree to which the leader is clinically knowledgeable and competent directly influences feelings of security about the appropriateness of nursing activity.*

Nurses have a responsibility to the client or his audience (see Chapter 1), to their employers, and to those being led to be clinically proficient. Clinical competence gives the nurse self-confidence, which is communicated in both tangible and intangible ways to clients, employers, and co-workers. Nurses who have sound basic knowledge and clinical expertise save time and energy for themselves and others. They understand when proceedings are correct, and they are more innovative in devising better ways to accomplish a given task. Clinically knowledgeable nurses are able to discuss with clients and care givers the validity of established goals, the appropriateness of planned activities, and the work schedule necessary for achieving those goals. Individuals who turn to the knowledgeable leader for help and advice are rewarded by having their needs met. This reinforces trust in the leader's competence and frees care givers to rely on themselves and on each other in cooperative efforts. Conversely, a group leader who engages in activities that do not contribute to goal accomplishment loses the confidence of the led and decreases the cooperative effort overall.

The nurse-leader who cleans the medication cupboard during the time allotted to the hygienic care of patients clearly establishes in the eyes of the group that his activities are not contributing to the accomplishment of nursing goals. The nurse-leader who allows group activity to become tangential to the goal also decreases effectiveness.

An example of tangential group activity is seen in the following:

Administration of nursing care is sidetracked by the failure of a hopper to function properly. Group efforts are focused on reestablishing proper functioning of the hopper, and group members spend their time in activities that are not goal oriented.

***

*Management and supervision of patient care, Nurs. Clin. North Am. 8:(2), June, 1973.

These activities may be rewarding and interesting for a time, but the members will soon become aware that the work assigned will have to be done whether the hopper functions properly or not. When the assigned work is not accomplished within the time alloted, the group loses confidence in the leader's ability to direct activity, which, in turn, results in loss of esteem. The effective leader would have reported the faulty plumbing and refocused group effort toward established goals. In this way the member's confidence in the leader would be reinforced by his ability to guide activity through unforeseen circumstances to successful achievement of goals.

MUTUAL RESPECT

Maximum productivity results when consideration and respect are given to a health care giver's total personality; this means that recognition and utilization of the employee's desires, attitudes, interests, and motives are as important as attention to his physical efforts.

As consideration for worth and respect of the individual has progressed in health agencies, many current practices have developed. These include a recognition that individuals vary in their personal aptitudes and interests, that different jobs require different abilities, that the emotional make-up of the individual influences job performance, and that the prevailing spirit or feeling of the work force affects productivity. The need for mutual respect between an employer and employee is gradually being recognized. Both have an interest in the well-being of the other, and the relationship between employer and employee must be harmonious if they are to work together toward their common objectives. This same philosophy applies to nurse-leaders and co-workers.

PREDICTIVE PRINCIPLE: *Understanding and practicing the basic elements of mutual respect facilitate effective leadership.*

Maximum utilization of personnel is influenced by the mutual respect between group and leader. Determination of basic elements inherent in respect is a difficult task in a society where people from varied backgrounds, free to develop their own philosophies of life, compose the work force.

In 1951 the National Education Association published the results of a survey to determine if there was a core of spiritual and moral values for operation in a free society upon which all people could agree. The following values were agreed upon:*

1. There is significance in the individual personality. (This was the basic assumption from which all others were formulated.)
2. The individual has the capacity to assume moral responsibility.
3. Institutions are the servants of men; men are not the servants of institutions.
4. Common consent is a basis for social action.
5. Devotion to truth is necessary for open, trusting human relationships.

---

*Educational Policies Commission: Moral and spiritual values in the public schools, Washington, D. C., 1951, National Education Association, pp. 17-34.

6. Excellence in human achievement should be respected.
7. Moral equality is mandatory. No one in a democratic society has the moral right to injure the growth and development of another personality.
8. There should be brotherhood among people. This means the concern of one person for another—the interest of all people in relation to each other.
9. The pursuit of happiness is a legitimate goal.
10. Spiritual enrichment is desirable.

These points were the consensus of representatives from all ethnic groups, creeds, and religions in America as values that could serve as a basis for interrelationships. If the nurse-leader accepts these values and believes there is significance, worth, and dignity in the human personality, behavior, and attitudes, this belief will be indicated to others, and respect will be reciprocal.

Team members invest authority in their nurse-leader with the expectation that their worth will be recognized and that the leader will attempt to meet their needs in the work situation and will support their values.

PREDICTIVE PRINCIPLE: *Expressions of respect for others by the leader precipitate acts of mutual respect among members.*

Nurse-leaders who care for others enter into relationships with co-workers that have significance and create feelings of mutual satisfaction and respect. When the practitioner's attitude indicates concern for co-workers, a respect model is provided. Knowledge of members' personal problems requires the nurse-leader to express feelings of concern and understanding and to construct a work environment that fosters the growth and potentialities of the members.

Situations can be structured that will enable members with problems to find ways within the work situation to deemphasize personal problems. However, it must be recognized that the nurse-leader's role is confined to prescribed activities within the work situation.

Admiration and respect for others can be expressed in many ways and still be in keeping with commitment. Sometimes the nurse-leader is hesitant to share feelings of esteem for others because of a fear that intentions will be misinterpreted or effectiveness as a leader will be lessened. The mature leader will realize the value of expressing feelings for others on appropriate occasions and will not deprive himself and others of the opportunity for successful reinforcement of positive relationships that comes from such expressions. A leader who respects another person will become involved in that person's development, and mutual growth will result.

Attitudes concern feelings and opinions and are revealed in both overt and covert ways. Those who are led expect the leader's attitudes to be constructive. They expect such attitudes as warmth, acceptance, objectivity, empathy, compassion, and respect to be exhibited by the leader. When the nurse-leader demonstrates to co-workers that others are held in high regard, a pattern of behavior for that group (feelings of trust) will be nurtured and mutual respect will follow. The nurse-leader and members will accept and respect one another as peers and work together to minimize weaknesses and maximize strengths.

When the concept of mutual respect is learned by the nurse-leader, constructive attitudes among members will be promoted. The extent to which coworkers adopt the nurse's attitudes toward others is a measure, to some degree, of the effectiveness of the leader.

OPEN CHANNELS OF COMMUNICATION

Many nurse-leaders feel unaffected by the environment in which they work. They are preoccupied with clients, audience, other members of the health team, or with the administrative staff of the area. Authority figures are frequently equated with punishment and discipline. No previous personal contact with a specific managerial person or position is necessary for the authority figure to cause anxiety in some nurses. Effective utilization of the administrative staff in an agency, of an independent practitioner, or a primary care giver presumes knowledge of the position and the function of each job and a broad understanding of the channels of communication.

PREDICTIVE PRINCIPLE: *Knowledge of appropriate channels of communication facilitates efficient utilization of line organization.*

The purpose of independent practitioners and health agencies is to provide quality health service to patients. This purpose is sometimes lost in the bureaucracy that has evolved in the struggle to meet rapidly expanding demands for health services, and the operation becomes an end in itself.

Nurses who know the lines of communication within and without formal health organizational structures can cope with the setting and can devise ways to facilitate and expedite nursing practice.

Studying the line organizational chart from an agency policy manual will not necessarily describe the responsibilities of each position. The nurse-leader needs to acquire knowledge not only of the line organization but also of job descriptions, if the organizational structure is to be useful.

The line organizational chart and the de facto organizational structure may not be the same; some people in the authority structure may be assuming roles and responsibility that has been officially prescribed to others. This can happen by incorrectly established custom or as a result of power struggles. The nurse-leader who participates in such practice reinforces the habit of working through inappropriate administrative personnel and is placed in a difficult and sometimes untenable position. When the nurse-leader finds that such conflicts exist, clarification should be sought from the nurse-leader's immediate superior in written form. Written memos empower the staff nurse to function more securely by providing a record of clarified channels for future reference.

Confusion, wasted energy, and decreased service to the patient as a result of poor use of the organizational structure can result in a situation such as the following:

> The nurse-leader asks the supervisor of the unit for permission to hold a class with the ancillary staff about colostomy care. The supervisor gives permission and encouragement. The staff nurse asks the director of central supply to demonstrate use of the equipment. The nurse then posts a notice in the dining room inviting all interested

nurses to attend. The in-service education director becomes upset because in-service education is his area of authority and he should have been consulted about the class.

The nurse-leader could have prevented problems in this situation by using the appropriate chain of command. Casual perusal of the organizational chart and job descriptions would have indicated to the nurse-leader that the in-service education director was a necessary person to consult before proceeding with plans involving other departments and people from other nursing units.

PREDICTIVE PRINCIPLE: *The nurse working in an expanded role provides leadership initiative in establishing channels of communication congruent with the role.*

The nurse engaged in collaborative interprofessional relationships, as in the practice of primary nursing care and/or expanded roles, will establish relevant and expedient channels of communication between employer, client and related individuals, or other implicated members of the health team. The expanded role includes persons and/or functions that contribute to the nurse's care giving repertoire. The practitioner establishes avenues of communication with these resources so that combined knowledge, skills, and support will be immediately assessable in routine or critical health giving situations. The expanded role requires the independent nurse to be conversant with contributing sources of communication and enables him to function appropriately in a given circumstance.

The nurse practitioner who functions beyond ordinary discipline boundaries performs without the structure often attendant with regulations of advisory councils, committees, and other direction-giving bodies. An expansion in role does not imply that the nurse is absolved from accountability to organizational framework whether casual (as with a verbal agreement between client and nurse) or highly structured (as in a complex health agency). Seeking suitable resources, guidance, and such other contributory assists that accrue from established policy and procedure, either within or without the health agency, contribute to the client's welfare and the nurse's professional development.

KNOWLEDGE OF PARTICIPANTS' CAPABILITIES

Since World War II, nursing has been deluged with ancillary workers, each with a different background and preparation. These workers enter the nursing field to perform selected tasks under the supervision and direction of professional nurses. They bring to the job a wide variety of sociocultural and educational backgrounds. Nurse-leaders who assess the capabilities of each individual with whom they work can delegate tasks and responsibilities appropriately and assist each worker in developing his potential.

PREDICTIVE PRINCIPLE: *An understanding of sociocultural backgrounds of members assists the leader to make an assessment of job capabilities.*

The recent advent of educational and training programs aimed at the unemployed and cultural and racial minority groups has brought large numbers of workers from various ethnic backgrounds into nursing. Race, English language skills, economic level, and the cultural experiences of these workers vary from the middle-class, white, third and fourth generation Americans that comprise the bulk of professional nurses. It is necessary that the nurse-leader be able to communicate clearly and relate effectively with these workers if their skills and knowledge are to be fairly assessed and their attitudes understood. This assessment helps the nurse-leader to understand the value systems (see Chapter 3) of group members, to know how best to motivate them, and thus to know how to communicate with them effectively. A value system is brought to the job as a part of each person's personality. An understanding of value systems enables the nurse-leader to use the entire work force to full advantage and to effectively promote the development of individual and group potential.

Barriers to understanding and rapport, such as race and class, are not insurmountable. Prejudice, caste, and class conflicts exist in nursing, as in society, both openly and subtly. However, because of the changing self-image of subcultural groups and the legal protection of individual rights and dignity, racial and class prejudices are discussed more freely today than ever before. Nurse-leaders who ignore the presence of a group member from a subculture or avoid talking about differences in cultural or ethnic background do not prevent conflict, they only drive it underground. The critical problems of today's society will be reflected in each small group and must be faced.

Open discussions about individual differences or similarities will enable a leader to recognize how cultural, class, or ethnic characteristics influence individual value systems and behavior patterns within the nursing group. Talking openly and directly about class, color, and culture is difficult for the average middle-class white nurse; however, success in this area will come with practice. An observant nurse-leader who is sensitive to others can remark upon incidents and solicit comments that help promote understanding of members. If a nurse-leader does not understand an individual's feelings, openly admitting the lack of understanding invites further exploration and leads to trust. Relationships based on understanding and insight promote the assessment of capabilities and the development of potential in individuals.

English language differences can influence how the leader perceives the care givers and can influence assessment of capabilities and potential. Dialects, poor grammar, foreign accents, and colloquial expressions along with unusual diction can mislead the unwary nurse-leader. Language differences are environmental, cultural, geographic, and educational; they have little to do with intelligence, ability, and job training. The effective nurse-leader will assess the worker's knowledge, maturity, skill, and experience, and avoid assumptions based on language alone.

PREDICTIVE PRINCIPLE: *Reactions to stress influence efficiency of performance in the work situation.*

Job capabilities are influenced by many factors other than ability, knowledge, and skill. Personal crises absorb energy and drain resources that would normally be utilized in work functions. Thought patterns and observational skills are interrupted or inhibited by preoccupation with personal crises. The skillful leader will observe departure from normal work patterns and try to ascertain the reasons for the altered performance. This knowledge enables the leader to change work assignments or supervisory habits to conform to the demands of the new behavior pattern until the personal crisis is past.

Stressful job situations, such as patient emergencies, unexpectedly heavy work assignments, breakdowns in communications and interrelationships, nursing errors, and conflicts with physicians or supervisors, elicit responses from the nurse-leader and other care givers that are not normally seen in daily routine behavior. The nurse-leader who knows each worker's behavioral patterns not only can help to prevent disruptions of client care but also can anticipate how best to help the distressed member. Opportunity for members to discuss stressful work factors and their feelings about them as soon after the incident as possible decreases the accompanying anxiety and allows the daily work to progress smoothly. Such discussions, while impressions and feelings are fresh, give all participants a truer picture of what actually happened and furnish insights that contribute to the leader's knowledge of individual capabilities, increase job satisfaction, and save time and energy.

PREDICTIVE PRINCIPLE: *Knowledge of a care giver's preparation and experience promotes fullest use of skills and provides a basis for continued growth.*

The nurse-leader needs specific information about the education and work experience of each group member to delegate the work load appropriately and to determine the amount of supervision and teaching necessary to develop personnel potential. Some of the necessary information may be in employment records, but frequently the personnel files are not open to staff nurses. The nurse is often dependent on personal interviews and observations for information necessary to proper utilization of all personnel. The following is an example:

> Mrs. Pedersen, a skilled nurse-leader, had worked with Mrs. Williams, an aide, for six months. Mrs. Pedersen discovered during a conversation at lunch one day that Mrs. Williams had worked in a home for the aged for 15 years. The aide stated that she had always loved aged people and liked to work with them; she derived satisfaction from getting them to eat and drink and from contriving ways to motivate them. Upon working with Mrs. Williams, Mrs. Pedersen observed that Mrs. Williams was very knowledgeable and creative with elderly patients and was able to learn much from working with her. As nurse-leader, Mrs. Pedersen utilized this aide to help other ancillary workers who were assigned to geriatric patients.

A formally planned assessment interview would have revealed Mrs. Williams' strength much earlier and would have benefited both patients and personnel.

Sources of information

Two basic sources of information are available to the nurse-leader—the personal interview and personal observation. The following outline is designed as a guide to activities that will provide the nurse-leader with needed member assessment data.

    I. The assessment interview
        A. Establishment of a time and place that provides privacy and freedom from interruptions
        B. Introduction of purposes of interview and how information will be used

C. Establishment of rapport conducive to an exchange of information; inquiring about the following to obtain the specific information desired:
  1. Educational background—amount of formal education (grade completed, high school diploma, post high school work, extent of college work)
  2. Formal job training
    a. Length of program and when completed
    b. Formal classroom content (anatomy and physiology; bacteriology and aseptic technique; talking with patients; procedures—list common ones encountered on present job; organization of work; observations—recording and reporting)
  3. Clinical practice
    a. Real or simulated situation (patient care or practice on dolls or fellow students)
    b. Experience in systems of care (primary, case, functional, team)
    c. Type of patients included in experiences (medical, surgical, obstetric, psychiatric)
    d. Nursing setting (home, convalescent hospital, acute hospital, out-patient clinics)
    e. Opportunity for practice of nursing procedures
    f. Amount of supervision
    g. Who supervised (teacher or nurse on unit or others)
    h. Nursing activity preferences and type of patients preferred
D. Conclusions
  1. Brief summary of notes taken regarding content and tone of interview
  2. Structure for follow-up at later date as necessary
II. Observation
  A. Observation of work in progress during normal work day activities
  B. Survey of work results
    1. Assignments completed as directed
    2. Patient appearance
    3. Content of reporting to group and nurse-leader and/or charting
  C. Observation of relationship with other personnel and group
  D. Participation observation

Assessment interview. Time and place for the assessment interview must be mutually convenient to both parties. A well-planned and structured interview does not take long. A prior explanation of what will occur in the interview should be given to the care giver so that he will come prepared and thus reduce the time required for the conference. Fifteen to 20 minutes should be sufficient for such an interview. Keeping appointments punctually and terminating the conference on time are important. Punctuality helps convey the value of both the worker's and the leader's time.

Setting an atmosphere for the interview occurs both during the preliminary discussions about the interview and within the interview itself. Openness and sincerity are behavioral messages that put the interview on an honest, productive basis. Subterfuge, hesitancy, and lack of candidness elicit responses with the same characteristics.

Nurse-leaders who ask co-workers, instead of the individuals involved, about fellow workers' abilities, problems, attitudes, and preparation are engaging in a practice that will create distrust among the members. Often, the leader who follows such a practice not only receives fallacious information but also loses the trust and support of the group.

A relaxed atmosphere is helpful to the establishment of rapport. Relaxed informality is not lack of structure; it is naturalness. Any activity, posture, or attitude that helps both parties behave in a normal way helps establish rapport. Both interviewee and the leader should feel free to smoke or take refreshment. These are socializing activities that promote naturalness. A room where there is privacy and, if possible, comfort is helpful. Job responsibilities of both persons should be assigned to other care givers for the duration of the interview; this enables the devotion of attention to the subject and prevents interruptions.

The nurse-leader who begins an interview with a well-defined plan for achieving objectives is likely to reach those objectives. Having a specific and topical list for discussion will produce the best results. Keeping the list in view and making notes as the interview progresses will be helpful to the interviewer by keeping attention focused on the subject and giving a brief record for future reference.

Evaluation of interview data requires sensitivity to nonverbal responses and interpretation of verbal responses. The nurse who fidgets, fusses, or verbally hedges may be attempting to say what he thinks the interviewer wishes to hear, to mask his true feelings, or to cope with anxiety. The interviewer must weigh all the responses (verbal and nonverbal) of the worker and attempt to evaluate them. Clarifying remarks can take the form of statements, observations, or questions, such as, "Will you describe what you learned in your classes on aseptic technique so that I understand a little better?" Statements calling for further descriptions, elucidation, and information help the nurse-leader to clarify and evaluate responses.

Observation. The leader must have practical and real knowledge of a group member's ability gathered from firsthand observations of the nurse at work. Assessment of the worker's ability can be made through several observational methods. Observing work in progress gives the leader insight into the worker's effectiveness, safety, and efficiency. Patients who appear clean and comfortable when care is completed and nursing care plans that have been carried through are indicators of worker ability. The content of written or oral reports can also be used by the nurse-leader as assessment data.

Participation-observation is probably the method of observing most effective for nurse-leaders. It will prove useful in assessments, which are done for the purpose of providing a basis for optimal utilization of personnel and encouraging professional growth. Participation-observation is observing another's conduct while participating with him in job performance, for example, observing how sheets are handled and how a bed is made while helping to make the bed. Participation-observation must be explained to ancillary workers to enable the nurse-leader to observe without usurping the worker's role. Participation-observation experiences provide the following opportunities:

1. An opportunity for the nurse-leader to assess the member
2. An opportunity for the nurse-leader to teach and learn
3. An opportunity for the nurse to observe the nurse-leader in the care of patients (role modeling)

Plans for participation-observations can be arranged in a group or meeting with the client or family in which the purposes for the observations are discussed. Arrangements can be made for the nurse-leader to work closely with each member at a convenient time. It is essential that the members have a clear understanding of the purposes of the participation-observation experiences.

Observational assessments help the nurse-leader to make assignments that enable the full utilization of each person's capabilities. Working together fosters mutual respect and mutual assessment. Since the nurse-leader has prescribed activities, plans must be made for short participation-observations on a daily basis so that observations can be made of routine work, as well as of special assignments or new procedures.

The ability to function is dynamic and changes with variables of conditions, environments, and associations with people. The nurse-leader can only try to assess and reassess each worker. This continuous assessment process enables the nurse-leader to delegate responsibility and supervise work appropriately while promoting the greatest development of personnel potential. The outcome of this approach will improve the quality and safety of nursing care.

ENVIRONMENT

The nurse-leader concentrates on human motivation and group behavior and takes into consideration the work environment, which in part determines the scope and limitations of activity.

Technical environment includes the physical geography, organizational layout, equipment, system of supply, scheduling, and methods of administering services. The nurse-leader's work environment includes all technical aspects and the conditions, circumstances, and pressures that influence administrative processes.

The findings of much of the research in executive behavior support the conclusion that effective performance of leaders is directly related to the organizational environment.

An alert and interested nurse-leader will find ways to meet personal needs in the work environment, protecting client, employees, and self from harmful environmental factors, taking advantage of desirable aspects, and changing the environment in ways that make it a better source of need satisfaction. To accomplish this, the nurse-leader understands and is able to apply those principles that contribute to a satisfactory environment.

PREDICTIVE PRINCIPLE: *A work environment that is open and amenable to valid change assists in personal and professional growth and development.*

Work experiences that allow the nurse-leader to satisfy intellectual curiosity enable an acquisition of skills and knowledge necessary for intelligent, efficient work and informed living.

Each leader and participant needs opportunities to engage in experiences that promote ongoing motivation to grow professionally. Work environments can make provision for the expression of personality through creative activities. Identification with the results of one's own activity and taking pride in personal achievements promote professional productivity. Creativity is seen at all levels and can be applied to the most ordinary tasks. Creativity that is utilized can increase efficiency. With imaginative design and innovation, job activities may be completed in less time, with less energy expended, and with less equipment used.

Originality of thought can result in increased service to patients and greater job satisfaction. Creativity fluorishes in an environment where each worker feels that his ideas and opinions are received by leaders and peers and are given the same consideration as every other group member's. Henry Ford believed that if a lazy man is given a job to do he will find the quickest and easiest way to perform the task. In the same vein, give a well-prepared nurse-leader a job, and he will devise the best possible way to perform the assignment.

It is possible to pursue the goals of individuals, organizations, and agencies without destroying human values in the process. The organization has a great stake in developing its people and thus in serving human values and organizational ends. Individual or small employers and management of health agencies that take specific steps to ensure the work environment gives nurse-leaders an opportunity to grow and develop will have more stable and productive personnel. The achievement of emotional maturity in the leader is dependent on an environment that provides him with opportunities to express independence and autonomy, to have a part in determining the outcome of efforts, and to participate in significant relationships with others. Innovations that promote desired changes in environment can support optimism and the freedom to be productive.

APPLICATION OF PREDICTIVE PRINCIPLES OF LEADERSHIP BEHAVIOR

In the role of primary care giver, the nurse assessed the geriatric, bed-rest client to be suffering from respiratory insufficiency.

PROBLEM	PRINCIPLES	PRESCRIPTION
The need for reduction or alleviation of respiratory insufficiency.	Knowledge of theory levels and ability to formulate valid predictive principles promote the leader's ability to identify the levels on which members are functioning to facilitate growth in problem solving and goal attainment. Knowledge of a care giver's preparation and experience promotes fullest use of skills and provides a basis for continued growth.	Proceed through four levels of theory building: 1. Name and categorize the problems (complete with assessment of problem). 2. Relate the factors (signs and symptoms) to normal base lines. 3. Relate to situation; e.g., recumbency and immobility lead to systemic tissue hypoxia and venous stasis; gravity makes mechanical resistance to breathing greater in the supine position than in the erect position. 4. Prescription: check lab results of blood gases, reorder if necessary; assess level of orientation, extent of knowledge, and willingness to participate in the development of a problem-oriented care plan; teach patient necessary knowledge and skills; plan with him times to elevate head; auscultate lungs for rales; cough, turn, and deep

Continued.

PROBLEM	PRINCIPLES	PRESCRIPTION
		breathe; observe rate, depth, and quality of respirations; passive range of motion exercises to extremities.
		Enlist support of client's family and other involved persons in carrying out care plan.

BIBLIOGRAPHY

BOOKS

Argyris, C.: Management and organizational development, New York, 1971, McGraw-Hill Book Co.

Auld, M. E., and Birum, L. H.: The challenge of nursing, a book of readings, St. Louis, 1973, The C. V. Mosby Co.

Barrett, H. H.: Individual goals and organizational objectives, a study of integration mechanisms, Ann Arbor, Mich., 1970, Institute for Social Research, The University of Michigan Press.

Brown, E. L.: Nursing reconsidered: a study of change. Parts 1 and 2. Philadelphia, 1970, J. B. Lippincott Co.

Carlson, C. E.: Behavioral concepts and nursing intervention, Philadelphia, 1970, J. B. Lippincott Co.

Combs, A. W., Avila, D. L., and Purkey, W. W.: Helping relationships, basic concepts for the helping professions, Boston, 1971, Allyn & Bacon, Inc.

Dolan, J. A.: Nursing in society, a historical perspective, Philadelphia, 1973, W. B. Saunders Co.

Guinée, K. K.: The professional nurse: orientation, roles, and responsibilities, New York, 1970, The Macmillan Co., Publishers.

Jourard, S. M.: Disclosing man to himself, Princeton, N. J., 1964, D. Van Nostrand Co.

Jourard, S. M.: The transparent self, Princeton, N. J., 1964, D. Van Nostrand Co.

Lewis, E. P.: Changing patterns of nursing practice: new needs, new roles, New York, 1971, The American Journal of Nursing Co.

Lysaught, J. P., editor: National Commission for the Study of Nursing and Nursing Education: an abstract for action, New York, 1970, McGraw-Hill Book Co.

Mager, R. F., and Pipe, P.: Analyzing performance problems, Belmont, Calif., 1970, Fearon Publishers.

Mager, R. F.: Goal analysis, Belmont, Calif., 1972, Fearon, Publishers.

Maslow, A. H.: Motivation and personality, New York, 1954, Harper & Row, Publishers.

PERIODICALS

Bingham, G.: Developing staff and records where traditional roles are changing, J. Nurs. Admin. pp. 36-47, Feb.-March, 1973.

Bradner, P.: A matter of identity, Nurs. Outlook 21(5):332-334, 1973.

Driscoll, V.: Liberating nursing practice, Nurs. Outlook 20(1):24-27, 1972.

Fagin, C.: Accountability, Nurs. Outlook 19(4): 249-251, 1971.

Ganong, W. L., and Ganong, J. M.: Reducing organizational conflict through working committees, J. Nurs. Admin. pp. 12-19, Jan.-Feb., 1972.

Greenidge, J., Zimmern, A., and Kohnke, M.: Independent group nursing practice: community practitioners—a partnership, Nurs. Outlook 21 (4):228-231, 1973.

Hall, D. T., and Nougaim, K. E.: An examination of Maslow's need hierarchy in an organizational setting, organizational behavior and human performance, Nurs. Outlook 16(3): 12-16, 1968.

Hartwig, M. S.: Role and identity: an important decision, Nurs. Outlook 20(1):665-669, 1972.

Miller, D. I.: Leaders march to a different drummer, J. Nurs. Admin. p. 3, Jan.-Feb., 1971.

Rafferty, C. J.: Nursing Consultations, Inc.—a corporation, Nurs. Outlook 21(4):232-235, 1973.

Rogers, M. E.: Nursing: to be or not to be? Nurs. Outlook 20(1):42-46, 1972.

Schweer, M. E., and Gardella, F. A.: Planning, Orienting and preparing for a new kind of nurse leadership, Nurs. Outlook 18(5):42-46, 1970.

Thomas, L. A.: Predicting change in nursing values, J. Nurs. Admin. pp. 50-58, May-June, 1971.

Walsh, M. E.: On nursing's role in health care delivery: some comments on the subject from NLN's general director, Nurs. Outlook 20(9): 592-593, 1972.

Appendix

DERIVATION OF PREDICTIVE PRINCIPLES FROM SEVERAL AUTHORITATIVE SOURCES

Principles are derived from events. People observe events and record the logical serial order of the occurrence of the event. A theory is established about the cause and effect of the event, which then must be tested for validation. If a theory or hypothesis can be validated, it becomes a law; if it cannot be validated, but evidence seems to support the theory, it is still a usable tool.

The nurse-leader is seldom the originator of a completely new fact, concept, law, or principle. In most instances the nurse-leader depends on the published work of authorities to provide the sources from which predictive principles may be extracted. Those who would compile predictive principles of any given topic must search the literature for pertinent material, critically evaluate the validity of the material, and convert the concepts gleaned from the literature into predictive principles. This process can be described in nine steps. The following are the operational steps in extracting predictive principles from the literature:

1. Determine the topic or area to be considered.
2. Search the literature for books, articles, or pamphlets germane to the subject.
3. Read extensively in the field; keep a list of frequently recurring concepts (and include the source of each concept for reference).
4. Identify in the literature statements about how concepts influence or are related to each other and make appropriate notations on the cumulative list.
5. Select from the accumulated list material relevant to the concept of the circumstances, conditions, or behaviors (CCB) triad.
6. Determine from the authoritative sources on the accumulated list the predicted outcome of the CCB triad concept selected.
7. Determine the appropriate active verb phrase that will connect the concepts selected.
8. Add the qualifiers that will precisely indicate the specific delineations necessary to make the predictive principle valid and relevant.
9. Repeat steps 5, 6, 7, and 8 for each additional predictive principle for the determined topic until all major concepts on the list have been formulated into predictive principles.

The following is an example of the extraction of one predictive principle from an authoritative source using the first eight steps.

PROBLEM: To make progressive changes in the nursing team routine.

1. *Determine the topic or area to be considered.* The topic is determined by the problem to be solved. In any given problem it will be necessary to use predictive principles from several areas. In this instance the nurse-leader would draw on a variety of topics or areas for predictive principles to use to accomplish the desired goals. Some of these areas would be leadership, teaching-learning, group dynamics, and interpersonal relationships. From each of these areas the nurse-leader would select or formulate the appropriate predictive principles for the task and designate them as "principles for making changes." This topic then becomes the area of desired predictive principles.

2. *Search the literature for books, articles, or pamphlets germane to the subject.* The objective for the review is to identify and extract those concepts which will form the basis for activities and behaviors that will stimulate and enable group change. The searcher seeks any resources that he postulates will be helpful in the determined subject area. For the above objective the nurse-leader would search the literature of such fields as psychology, sociology, business and industry, education, and nursing.

3. *Read extensively in the field; keep a list of frequently recurring concepts (including sources).* Certain topics or concepts recur with frequency in the literature of any given subject. A list of the recurring concepts enables the nurse-leader to determine the salient themes in any given subject with minimum effort and maximum speed. A list for the selected topic would contain such concepts as the objective of change, motivation, need, problem identification, group involvement, group commitment, individual security, careful planning, design and sequence for change, and optimum pace.

4. *Identify in the literature statements about how concepts influence, or are related to, each other, making appropriate notations on the cumulative list.* These notations are for the purpose of clearfying concept relationships and will readily facilitate the formulation of principles. The following is a cumulative list of concepts with notations that clarify concept relationships.

Concepts	*Notations about predicted outcome and relationships*
1. Clearly establish objectives of change	1. Direction, evaluation, minimum side-tracking
2. Group involvement	2. Related to commitment to outcomes of change
3. Group commitment	3. Grows with increasing participation in planning and decision-making
4. Individual security	4. Providing individual with knowledge and skills and right to err with ego support during change
5. Careful planning	5. Logical order, central authority
6. Design and sequence	6. Purpose, focus, pace, progress, individual security, limitations
7. Optimum pace	7. Imposed by time and available materials
8. Motivation	8.
9. Need	9.
10. Problem identification	10.

The list is incomplete as there are no notations for concepts 8, 9, and 10. The investigator need only follow the prescribed outline. Bibliographic data must be kept during the task so that credit may be given to the sources used.

5. *Select from the accumulated list material relevant to the concept of the CCB triad.* If the concept list and notations are complete, this step requires only that the appropriate concept be selected from the list. For example, "design and sequence" might be selected as the CCB triad concept.

6. *Determine from the authoritative sources or the accumulated list the predicted outcome of the CCB triad concept selected.* Again, as above, if the concept list and notations are complete, this step requires only that the appropriate predicted outcome be selected from the notations on the list. For example, the principle formulator selects "purpose," "focus," and "progress" from the alternatives on the compiled list.

With the CCB triad and the predicted outcome concepts selected, all that remains is to relate them in some logical, meaningful way.

7. *Determine the appropriate active verb phrase that will connect the concepts selected.* The active verb is important because it determines the extent and degree of the relationship between the CCB triad and the predicted outcome. The writer of the principle could choose words such as *ensure, influences,* or *promotes* for the active verb.

The principle formulator has found evidence in the literature that **purpose, focus,** and **progress** are influenced by many factors in addition to **design and sequence.** With this evidence in mind, the formulator selects "promotes" rather than "ensures" as a more valid active verb.

At this point in the construction of a predictive principle, the components appear as follows:

CCB triad	*Active verb*	*Predicted outcome*
Design and sequence	promote	purpose, focus, and progress

Although stated as a principle, qualifiers are needed to give the concepts context and limitations.

8. *Add the qualifiers that will precisely indicate the specific delineations necessary to make the predictive principle valid and relevant.* This is the final step in constructing a single principle. The choice of articles, adjectives, adverbs, and other parts of speech that set its limits is important because qualifiers affect the predictive principle's validity and clarity and may be necessary to make the predictive principle a complete sentence. A predictive principle using the above selected components complete with qualifiers could read as follows:

A carefully predetermined **design and sequence** for change **promotes** work that is **purpose focused** and **progress** that proceeds as rapidly as possible.

DERIVATION OF A PREDICTIVE PRINCIPLE FROM A SINGLE AUTHORITATIVE SOURCE

The writer of predictive principles may find a paragraph in an authoritative source clearly stating a predictive principle within the text itself. The predictive principle formulator will find it expedient to identify the parts of the predictive principle and extract it directly from the literature. Such a paragraph is quoted below, and the components of the predictive principle are identified within the text.

> Attaching the label of evolutionary to change might be viewed by some as an opportunity to forestall any real innovation or as an excuse for lack of progress. To the contrary, although the suggested pace is less rapid, *evolutionary change requires a carefully predetermined* **design** *with* **definite sequence,** *pace and substance. These considerations are necessary to* **insure** *that* **purpose** *is always centrally* **focused** *and* **progress accomplished** *with all deliberate haste.*[*]

In the above quotation the concept of the CCB triad stands out clearly as **"design with definite sequence."** The predicted outcome appears within the text as **"purpose . . . focused and progress accomplished."** The critical principle formulator will find **"insure"** unacceptable as a valid active verb and will substitute a more realistic one such as *promotes.* The result is a predictive principle derived directly from an authoritative source. It will read as follows:

> A carefully predetermined design and sequence for change promotes work that is purpose focused and progress that proceeds with deliberate haste.

COMMON PREDICTIVE PRINCIPLE FORMULATION ERRORS

Blunders or errors in predictive principle formation have some similarity to principles and are often confused with predictive principles. Discriminating between predictive principles and nonprinciples is often difficult. Familiarity with common errors in predictive principle formation can prevent misconceptions, reinforce valid examples, and help the beginner to avoid errors. Most common errors in predictive principle formation take the form of directions, descriptions, statements of fact, or pseudoprinciples. Below are examples of common errors in principle construction using the predictive principle stated previously.

Directions. Directions either state how to do something step by step or contain the words *should* or *ought to.* These are actually level IV situation-producing theories.

The effective leader should do the following:

1. Gather data pertinent to the current situation
2. Decide which data are applicable
3. Use data to make decisions

Descriptions. Descriptions state how a person behaves or what an activity is like. Descriptions often take the form of characteristics; there is no *active* verb.

> A good leader will always have knowledge pertinent to the current situation on which to base decisions and judgment.

Facts or valid statements. Facts or valid statements are usually about the circumstances, conditions, or behaviors, or about the predicted outcome; however, they do not show relationship.

> Knowledge is of use only if it is pertinent to the current problem.

Weak predictive principles take the form of principles in that they have a

---

[*]From Beggs. D. W.: Team teaching, Indianapolis, 1964, Unified College Press, Inc., pp. 102-103.

CCB triad connected to a predicted outcome; however, the active verb lacks the quality of certainty. Such words as *apparently, might, may,* and *perhaps* make the predictive so weak that it is almost useless as an action base.

> Leaders who have knowledge pertinent to the current situation might make valid judgments and decisions.

Invalid principles. Invalidity is the most common form of error. Predictions that use erroneous material or fail to use modifiers appropriately often produce invalid predictions.

Index